As I Walked with My Mother

by
Lucille Engro DiPaolo

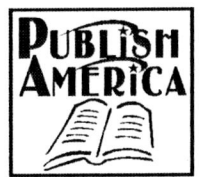

PublishAmerica
Baltimore

ISBN: 1-4241-0369-X
PUBLISHED BY PUBLISHAMERICA, LLLP
www.publishamerica.com
Baltimore

Printed in the United States of America

This book is dedicated to my husband Dom
for his unending love and support

I shall pass through this world but once.
Any good that I can do, or any kindness
that I can show to any living creature,
let me do it now, for I shall not pass this way again

Etienne DeGrellet

Table of Contents

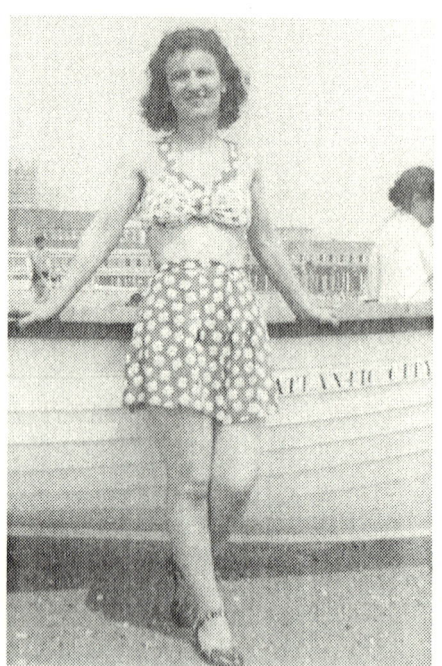

Fran in Atlantic City

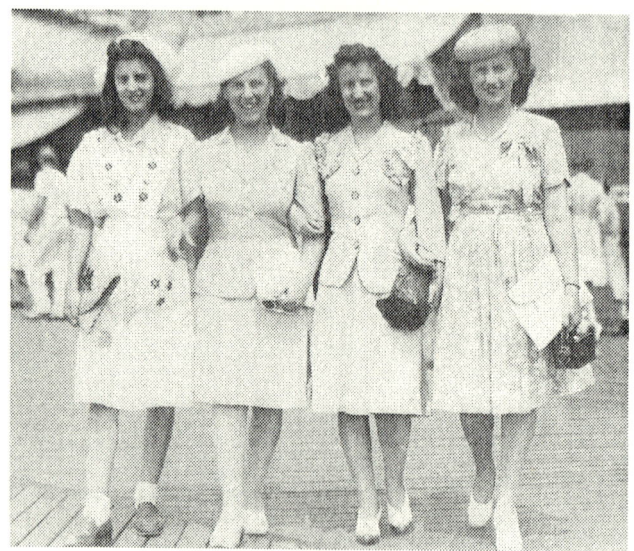

Atlantic City Boardwalk
Anne, Mary, Fran, and Florence

Introduction

As I Walked With My Mother is my experience in caring for my mom who suffered from Alzheimer's disease for three and a half years. Throughout this journey, I touch on our mother-daughter relationship as we go through a roller coaster of emotions in the final years of my mother's life.

I remember the day I walked into Mom's apartment to take her to the mall. She was waiting with a very angry look on her face.

"WELL, IT'S ABOUT TIME. DID YOU GET LOST?" she snapped.

"What do you mean? I came as soon as we hung up," I said.

"LIKE HELL YOU DID! I BEEN WAITING HERE ALL DAY!" she yelled.

I now looked at my mother and did not recognize her. Who was this angry woman? Who kidnapped my mother and left this impostor? She vaguely resembled her. I suddenly felt very sorry for myself.

That day I realized I lost my mother—the wonderful woman who loved and cared for me all of my life. The person who shared my joys and comforted me through my disappointments no longer existed. My best friend and confidante was gone. I was exhausted, bitter, and sad. I needed to vent my frustrations. But who would listen to me? Then I broke down and cried for my loss. I grieved because I no longer had a mother.

"I want my mother back," I sobbed. "I want my mother back."

Over four million Americans currently suffer from Alzheimer's disease. In the next decade that number is expected to skyrocket by 350 percent as America's baby boomers age. Caring for a loved one who is afflicted with this disease can be physically and emotionally draining. Studies have shown that caregivers themselves often become depressed and ill.

Alzheimer's disease intrudes on a person and family like an unwelcome stranger. This illness is not a sudden intrusion; it gradually makes its presence known and may last anywhere from three to twenty years. The vast majority of people experiencing memory problems are living at home but are not pursuing help. In the beginning stages, many families are in denial. They do not seek help until the disease progresses to a more advanced stage when it is impossible to ignore.

As I Walked With My Mother evolved as I gathered information about dementia and experienced the personality changes of a loved one afflicted with Alzheimer's disease. Through this journey with my mom, I share my coping skills as I learn to deal with emotions such as anger, sadness, guilt, and fear. I give practical tips that may be helpful to any family member dealing with the care of a memory-impaired patient. Every family affected will have its own unique situation.

Therefore, it is important to recognize this illness and get a diagnosis as soon as possible. Start with a complete physical examination from the primary physician. Other conditions can cause memory lapses and mental confusion. A physical exam could rule out other possibilities. The primary physician may then refer the patient to a specialist on aging to conduct necessary tests and to determine if the illness is Alzheimer's. Becoming familiar with the challenges of this type of dementia could minimize a crisis. I found that the early phase of this disease was the most troublesome because I did not know what was happening to my mother. If you understand this illness early, it becomes easier to make the necessary adjustments.

Unfortunately, Alzheimer's disease is often characterized in very dismal terms. When your loved one is initially diagnosed, it is easy to experience feelings of doom. We tend to stereotype victims of Alzheimer's with being in the late stages of the disease—people without any quality to life. This very grim image of a completely helpless individual may never become a reality.

When my mother was first diagnosed with Alzheimer's, I, too, saw this as an ongoing tragedy. I believed there could be no positive results from my hard work. Initially, my response to this stress was fear, anger, and depression. This left me depleted of energy. Despair was an everyday reality, and I felt as though I was suffering through an endless funeral.

However, my attitude changed when I started to perceive this situation as an opportunity to grow and add meaning to my life. When I thought of being a caregiver as my purpose or mission in life, I was able to contend with the difficult situations better. I accepted the limits that dementia imposed on my mother but realized there was growth potential with each encounter. I decided to accept this as a challenge instead of being confronted with insurmountable problems. There still were frustrating days but when I stopped being angry at what fate put before me, caregiving became an enriching experience. Dealing with Alzheimer's brought out a strength that I did not know I possessed.

I have learned an important lesson. There is no right or wrong way of handling the situation because the illness will affect every person differently. Even the same person's reaction will vary on different days. Many times it is trial and error. A characteristic of Alzheimer's is the gradual changes in an affected person as the illness becomes more pronounced. A caregiver may come up with a plan that works but must always be ready to look for a new approach. Throughout this book, I have written about strategies and guidelines that I found helpful.

Watching my mother struggle with Alzheimer's and old age gave me a better appreciation for life. I have become aware of the passing of time. As part of the baby boomer generation, I now face my own mortality and wonder what my health challenges will be in the not too distant future. However, I refuse to dwell on this. Instead I strive to improve and maintain my health and then concentrate on the positives.

As I Walked With My Mother depicts precious moments of our mother-daughter bond when Mom was the center of our family, and we depended on her. Also, there are times of the role reversal in our relationship.

Family members struggling with the care of a loved one suffering from dementia may benefit from reading about my experience. You have a tremendous responsibility to make sure that your loved one lives life to the fullest. At the same time, you must stay centered in spite of the sacrifices you will make. It is important to realize that you cannot give more than you have.

In the three and a half years that my mother struggled with her memory loss, I helped her maintain quality to life. This caregiving experience brought forth in me a personal resiliency and an intense determination. Being the primary caregiver for my mother during her final years is one of my most meaningful accomplishments.

1
Overview of Alzheimer's

Dementia is the "disease of the century." It is various disorders, which affect mental losses in multiple areas such as memory, language, and the ability to solve problems in daily life. The most common form of dementia is Alzheimer's disease. Today more and more people are receiving the heartbreaking news that the older members of their families have Alzheimer's disease. It is especially difficult to watch the mental deterioration of a parent who once was the center of the family. This illness usually affects people over the age of 60 and destroys their remaining years. It attacks people regardless of gender, ethnicity, or socioeconomic circumstance. However, statistics show that Alzheimer's disease afflicts more women. This might be because women outlive men by seven to twelve years.

A recent survey estimated that 4.5 million people in the United States over the age of 65 suffer from Alzheimer's.[1] Age is the greatest risk factor for this illness. One in 10 individuals over the age of sixty-five and nearly half over eighty-five are affected.[2] With our advanced technology, stronger antibiotics, and better health care, Americans are living longer. People 85 years of age and older represent the fastest-growing age group in our population. The birth rate remains low, and the size of the population over 65 is steadily increasing.

Alzheimer's could strike a person in his or her 30's or 40's. When symptoms of Alzheimer's appear before 60, this is considered early-onset Alzheimer's disease. The main difference between the two forms of the disorder is the way it affects the lives of a younger person as opposed to the older individual. While cognitive impairment is devastating at any age, the younger person is faced with having to quit his or her job. It is especially sad when the impaired individual has family responsibilities such as caring for children. This is a rare inherited form of the disease that has been linked to a specific gene.[3]

Alzheimer's disease has been called the "silent epidemic" that destroys human brains and diminishes the victims to a helpless state. This epidemic was described as silent because until recently very little was known about Alzheimer's.

Alois Alzheimer, a German neurologist identified the illness in 1906, but doctors did not study it seriously until the 1960s. Until that time, people assumed that confusion and memory loss were a natural part of aging. It was considered an inevitable part of growing old. However, it is not the fate of every elderly person. Medical experts believe that it is normal for older people to experience some problems with memory. When a person is diagnosed with Alzheimer's disease, he or she experiences severe, progressive memory loss and confusion. These are symptoms from a destructive disease that actually cause physical damage to the brain.

Alzheimer's disease is not easy to diagnose because its symptoms are very similar to other illnesses affecting the brain. Patients who have a number of small strokes (Multi-Infarct Dementia) appear to have clinical features similar to those of Alzheimer's. Some patients suffering from Parkinson's disease may exhibit the same cognitive changes. Also, depression can be confused with Alzheimer's disease because a depressed person could become extremely apathetic. Therefore, he or she could seem cognitively impaired.

The simplest way for doctors to determine whether a patient is suffering from Alzheimer's is to eliminate the other dementing illnesses. A physician needs to know about the general health and habits of the patient: Does the patient have diabetes or high blood pressure? Could there be a possible misuse of medications? Does the patient heavily use alcohol? Could the patient be suffering from a head injury?

Also, the patient needs to undergo blood tests and urinalysis. An EEG will indicate brain damage caused by a stroke or tumor but **not** damage caused by Alzheimer's. A special x-ray was designed called *Cat scanning* which is somewhat helpful in diagnosing Alzheimer's. The **CAT** scans often show shrinkage of the brain tissue that result when lesions of Alzheimer's disease are destroying cells. Although **CAT** scans can be helpful in diagnosing this disease, it should not be used alone to make a positive diagnosis.

There is a more advanced scan that is becoming a major diagnostic technique in determining the presence of neurological conditions. This is called the **PET** scan where blood flow in the brain can be measured. This technique involves injecting the patient with radioactive tracers.

PET scanning shows vivid images of the brain. There is a distinctive difference in the image that appears in the part of the brain that is affected by Alzheimer's. The **PET** scan is also useful in determining different forms of dementia such as epilepsy, Parkinson's, and Huntington's disease. With the **PET** scan, the damage in the brain can be seen in the very early stages.[4] There is still no cure for Alzheimer's but diagnosing a patient with the disease early on will enable the victim to start effective therapy.

An **MRI** technique called arterial spin labeling has been accurate in distinguishing Alzheimer's from frontotemporal dementia (FDA), according to a new study at San Francisco VA Medical Center.[5] FDA is a degenerative condition affecting the front part of the brain; Alzheimer's affects the hippocampus and the temporal lobe. The two conditions exhibit similar symptoms in the beginning stages but have different characteristics in the later stages. It is important to have an accurate diagnosis so the proper treatment can be given. Norbert Schuff, Ph.D a researcher at SFVAMC feels this technique has the potential to distinguish other types of dementia.

Scientists continue to study this devastating illness, and new diagnostic methods are being researched. Researchers at Northwestern University did a study that can detect microscopic amounts of toxic protein that may be responsible for early neurological deterioration in the Alzheimer's patient. This test is called **BCA** bio-bar-code amplification.[6]

Unfortunately, the patient suffering from memory impairment is not the only victim. Most people with some form of dementia live at home and are cared for by family members. This could cause a great emotional, physical, and financial strain on the family. Because of the potential long-term burden, family members are recognized as the secondary victims of Alzheimer's disease.

Before 1974, there was a tendency to disregard people who showed signs of senility. The feeling was that this affliction was untreatable and incurable. Since that time, the Alzheimer's Disease and Related Disorders Association (ADRDA) have made great strides in raising consciousness about Alzheimer's disease. Also after our former President Ronald Reagan was diagnosed with Alzheimer's, the Reagan Research Institute was established. The goal of this private sponsored research institute is "to accelerate the discovery and development of treatment and prevention for Alzheimer's disease by increasing information exchange, technology transfer, and alliance among investigators."

A study funded by the Elan Corporation and Wyeth Ayerst Laboratories shows some promise.[7] This entails vaccinating people to fight against Alzheimer's disease as we did for illnesses such as polio and smallpox. It involves injecting a person with the plaque causing beta-amyloid protein that is thought to be responsible for this disease. In the controlled group, twenty percent of the vaccinated people developed antibodies to the plaque. This suggests that the immune system could attack this amyloid protein and clear out the plaque that would prevent this brain-wasting disease from progressing or developing. Research holds hope and promise for the future.

Alzheimer's disease is no longer considered the natural consequence of living to an advanced age. Like any other disease, it is now subjected to scientific research. This leaves us with the hope that Alzheimer's will be curable in the future.

2
At the Graveside

The day was unusually mild for December. I didn't even need a coat as I stood with my husband at my mother's graveside among my relatives and friends. My father was standing to the right of me shaking and completely devastated. I always pictured my dad as a husky truck driver and a decorated World War II hero. I look at him now and see a broken man with no desire to go on living. I barely recognize him.

When did he get so old? I thought.

My parents were married for almost 54 years. Up until the last three years, Mom took care of him. Besides taking care of everything in the house, Dad even depended on her to tell him what to wear and to remind him to take his medicine. They both had their roles in life and never wanted to grow with the times. They were so comfortable with familiarity and took each other for granted. When Mom could no longer take care of these things, I took over, but Mom was still there. The last couple days, Dad appeared to be in a state of disbelief, especially when he looked at Mom's empty chair. With all his health problems, Dad always felt he was going to go first.

I then whispered to the undertaker, "Could you get my dad a chair before the prayer ritual starts? I'm afraid he is going to collapse."

"Oh sure," he said. He was back in a few minutes with a chair.

"Thanks," I said politely, and we got Dad seated.

Then I wondered why I had to take care of these little details on a day like this? For the last three years, it feels as if I had been doing the thinking for Mom and Dad, and now it was becoming habit forming.

The priest was reciting prayers. I tried to focus on the moment, but my mind kept wandering. When Father mentioned the deceased name, Frances Engro, I became a bit startled.

Is my mother really in that casket? Are we really going to put her in the ground?

Then I glanced at my brother. Chuckie has severe Down's Syndrome.

I wonder how much of this he understands. What does he feel? I hope he doesn't think that our mother who loved him so much throughout his life has deserted him.

Mom always worried about Chuckie.

"Who will watch over 'My Chuckie' when I'm gone?" she would say with a tear caught in her throat.

I had gone back and forth in my mind for the last three days deciding whether Chuckie should be present for this. I decided he should be here. I asked Wayne, the supervisor of the group home where my brother lives, if he would stay with Chuckie and tend to his needs for the day. If it looks as if it is too uncomfortable for Chuckie, Wayne was there to take him away from the situation.

I continued to stand there very calmly and in control. I do not remember crying at all that day. I was so calm that the people around me thought it was odd. In fact, it seemed a bit odd even to me. Everyone knows that I am extremely sensitive and emotional—sometimes to a fault. I have been known to cry at a touching commercial. When I went to see the movie Forrest Gump, I came out of the theater with an excruciating headache because I tried for two hours to hold back the tears.

When my friend Sandy's mother passed away, I left the funeral home feeling heartsick. I remember stopping the car on the side of the road because the tears were blinding my eyes. I also remember feeling fortunate that my mother was still very healthy, but a thought crossed my mind. How will I ever deal with losing Mom? Perhaps my tears were for the future loss of my mother.

I always had an extremely close relationship with Mom. She shared my joys and comforted me through my disappointments. Through the years, we laughed together; at times we became angry and frustrated, but no one will ever love me unconditionally like Mom.

With that kind of love and closeness that my relatives and friends knew I shared with my mother, no one expected me to stand here today without showing emotion. The only way I could explain it is I mourned my mother's passing for three years. As her mind slowly slipped away, she became more and more dependent on me. I grieved for my loss at different times with each episode caused by Alzheimer's disease. Gradually I mourned a living person whom I took care of and nurtured daily.

At first, my grieving was imperceptible. It had been a slow process of denial, acknowledgment, acceptance, and then finally disengagement. Mom was no longer the person with whom I shared my feelings. She became my dependent. Since she did everything for my father most of their married life, he also became my dependent. Fortunately, Chuckie was doing well living in the group home, but I still felt the need to be his advocate so life would continue to go smoothly for him.

Many times during the course of this illness, I grieved for the loss of my mother. Now that her body finally followed, my mourning has almost ended.

3

First Sign

Our heads were bowed as the priest continued the prayer. I happened to look up and noticed my cousins Dolores, Eleanor, and Lois. I think the last time I saw them was when my uncle passed away. With the older family members dying, our family is getting very small. I am going to make an effort to stay connected with my cousins. Funerals make you realize how much you need family. Then I noticed my cousin Dave.

Dave always said, "Nobody makes pizza like Aunt Fran."

Mom never used a recipe, but I did make homemade pizza once with her. It was delicious, but I said, "I am not making this again. It is just too long and complicated." She made her own dough and picked the fresh tomatoes and onions from her garden. The things you think of at the oddest times.

THAT'S WHEN I NOTICED SOMETHING WAS NOT QUITE RIGHT! I was in Mom's kitchen. She wanted some Jell-O and got the box out of the cabinet. She looked a bit confused as she examined the box of Jell-O and was trying to figure out what to do.

"Mom, boil the water," I said impatiently. She still looked confused. "How is it that you don't know how to make Jell-O?" I said.

"I know how to make Jell-O," she retorted. "It's just that I haven't made it for a long time."

"Let me do it. It's real easy. See," I said as I dissolved the powder in the boiling water. Then we both started to laugh. How ridiculous it was that Mom was a bit confused on making Jell-O.

Then there was the day that we all went to Denise's graduation. Her first grandchild was graduating from college, and Mom was very proud and excited.

To add to our pride, Denise was going to medical school. The graduation ceremony at Moravian College was held outside. That day we were experiencing a heat wave. It had to be over 90 degrees. I came prepared carrying a huge cooler of water and paper cups. As we were seated waiting for the ceremony to begin, our group kept drinking water. I kept asking Mom, "Aren't you thirsty?"

"No, I'm fine," she said.

After a while I would ask again and got the same response. Finally I just poured a cup of water and said, "Mom, you better drink this. I can't believe you aren't thirsty."

In hindsight, I found out that losing your sense of thirst is a symptom of Alzheimer's.

It is difficult to pinpoint the exact time that dementia occurs. Usually the onset of Alzheimer's is so gradual that in the beginning it is not noticeable so it becomes easy to dismiss. The afflicted person may realize there is a problem with his or her memory and becomes skillful in concealing this. They use notes to jolt their memory and continue to do most of the chores he or she has always done.

Some individuals become angry and blame others for their mistakes. A person with mild memory impairment may realize there is a problem and even mention his or her faulty memory. Sometimes your loved one is aware of the grave situation and will want to participate in treatment and planning for his or her future.

4
Something Is Wrong

There is a fairly large crowd at the cemetery. I felt touched that so many people came to pay tribute to my wonderful mother. I glanced at the faces and recognized the Bono's, Hammond's, and Gallo's—all friends from the neighborhood where my mother grew up.

There is my cousin Gina. The last time I saw her was over three years ago at a family gathering. I remember Gina coming up to Mom.

"Aunt Fran, how you doing?"

Mom politely answered, "Fine, and how are you?" Mom looked a little puzzled and did not say much more to Gina. Then I chimed in, and Gina and I started to catch up on what was happening in our lives. When Mom and I walked away, I mentioned to Mom that she acted kind of rude. "Mom, do you know her?" I asked.

Mom shook her head no. "I can't quite place her."

"Mom, that's Gina, your niece," I said.

"That's Gina!" she exclaimed.

"Yep," I said.

"Oh for heaven sakes," she said with a bit of embarrassment. Mom did go back to talk to Gina and was her warm and loving self.

It seemed to me that too many of these incidents were occurring now. That week I made a doctor's appointment for Mom in spite of her objections.

"Mom, don't give me a hard time. There may be something that could be done," I said.

"There's nothing wrong with me!" she stated. **"I'm fine. You act like you never forget anything."**

I sat in the office with Mom that week as Dr. Weiss examined her.

"My daughter thinks I'm losing my mind," Mom said sarcastically.

I told the doctor of the changes in Mom and the most recent incident with Gina.

Mom jokingly said, "Well, how was I suppose to recognize her? I hadn't seen her in years. And besides that, she sure got fat!"

Dr. Weiss told me Mom was in great physical shape. Her blood pressure was good. She had lost some weight, but Mom always was weight conscious and did a lot of walking. Dr. Weiss said he did notice a bit of confusion. But she still maintained her sense of humor, which is a good sign. He said there are drugs that may help and wrote a prescription. After the doctor's appointment, we went out to breakfast at Jems. While sitting in the booth, I brought up the subject of her forgetfulness.

"Mom, I hope the pills help," I said cautiously.

"Oh, I don't need any pills," Mom adamantly stated.

It was going to be difficult to get Mom to take anything. She had been very healthy all of her life, and if she had any aches and pains, you never knew it.

"Mom, we've got to try something. You're eighty-four and…"

"I am not eighty-four," Mom interrupted. "I'm eighty-three," she corrected. "Don't make me older than I am."

Well she was right about that, even though she would be eighty-four in a couple weeks.

"But Mom, that's besides the point. The fact is your body is probably healthier than a lot of fifty-year-olds. You have a long life ahead of you so we need to stop the brain from aging," I stated.

At that point the waitress brought our breakfast, and we got off the subject. Mom did have a healthy appetite, but in hindsight she probably forgot to eat at times which is a sign of dementia.

As long as I could remember, my mother always snacked a lot, especially while she was cooking and cleaning. I rarely remember Mom sitting down and eating. She was always jumping up and down from the table to get something. Now that she was slowing down, Mom probably forgot to snack. My mother did take the pills. They may have slowed the progression of the disease slightly but were no cure.

5
Most Difficult Stage

Those months when Mom was in her first stage of Alzheimer's disease were the most difficult. In addition to being forgetful, Mom became so obstinate. She did not want any help with household chores. She did not like anyone telling her what to do. I wonder if Mom knew something was happening to her and was trying to hide it. It must have been so confusing and frightening.

Fortunately my parents sold their home years ago. That decision was mainly because of Dad's health problems. Now they lived in a nice little apartment. It would have been easy to help Mom clean the apartment if she would just let me. Every time I would clean, Mom got angry. It would take me so long to scrub the bathroom, only because Mom was constantly yelling and hanging on me.

"LEAVE IT ALONE. I'LL DO IT LATER!" she yelled.

"MOM, WHY CAN'T YOU JUST BE GLAD THAT I'M DOING IT FOR YOU?" I asked.

"BECAUSE I LIKE DOING IT MYSELF!" she angrily shouted.

When I would finish a chore, I was so exhausted mainly from the arguments. It was like pulling a toy away from a child. After a couple of these episodes, I learned to sneak in

28

her apartment when she wasn't there. That was hard because whenever she would go out, it was usually with me. I mentioned to Dad that he would have to drive Mom to the market so I could clean without interruption. It was so much easier, and I would get done quickly. When Mom and Dad would come home, she never mentioned her clean apartment. Did she actually believe she kept the place in order? Maybe she didn't even notice.

This lack of awareness is a blessing in disguise for victims of dementia. It protects them from comprehending the magnitude of the situation. It does become more burdensome for the caregiver when a loved one does not cooperate and acknowledge he or she needs help.

On some level, Mom must have realized she was having a memory problem. She was having trouble recognizing people whom she knew but hadn't seen for a while. But Mom still had enough cognitive ability to hide her forgetfulness. She was even trying to conceal it from me.

Once when Mom and I were at the mall, I happened to see an acquaintance of mine. We started talking for a few minutes when Mom came up and acted as if she knew the woman even though I knew Mom never met her.

"Hi, how have you been? You're looking good," Mom said.

The woman politely smiled as she said, "Thank you."

When we walked away, I asked Mom, "Do you know her?"

"Yeah I know her," Mom replied.

"What's her name?" I asked.

"I know her, but I just can't remember her name," Mom said with certainty.

"It's Linda," I said.

"Oh yeah, that's right. It's Linda," she stated.

Well, at least Mom has enough cognitive ability to devise ways of being sneaky.

Fortunately, my daughters Denise and Kristen were both independent. Dom had a good job, and we were doing well. I did not have to work but had an interesting, great paying part time job as a Theme Reader with Colonial School District. So at this stage of my life, I was able to maintain caring for my parents along with my own household and manage a job. I remember constantly being on the road driving from my house in Plymouth Meeting to Mom and Dad's apartment in West Norriton—sometimes twice a day.

I remember the day I walked into Mom's apartment to take her to the mall. She was waiting for me with a very angry look on her face.

"WELL, IT'S ABOUT TIME. DID YOU GET LOST?" she snapped.

"What do you mean? I came as soon as we hung up," I said.

"LIKE HELL YOU DID. I BEEN WAITING HERE ALL DAY," she yelled.

I now looked at my mother and did not recognize her. Who was this angry woman? Who kidnapped my mother and left this impostor? She vaguely resembled her. I suddenly felt very sorry for myself.

That day I realized I lost my mother—the wonderful woman who loved and cared for me all of my life. The person who shared my joys and comforted me through my disappointments no longer existed. My best friend and confidante was gone. I was exhausted, bitter, and sad. I needed to vent my frustrations. But who would listen to me? Then I broke down and cried for my loss. I grieved because I no longer had a mother.

"I want my mother back," I sobbed. "I want my mother back."

This was the first of many times that I grieved the death of my mother.

6
What Is Alzheimer's Disease

I did make an appointment with Dr. Pearlstein, a specialist for the elderly. Mom was given a series of tests only to confirm what we already knew. She was in the first stage of Alzheimer's disease. This is a progressive disease that has a degenerative effect on the brain causing severe dementia. The first signs of the disease are slight memory disturbance or subtle changes in personality such as irritability, anxiety and depression.

Also, as the disease progresses, other symptoms may occur such as sleep disturbances, restlessness, delusions, and hallucinations. Some people have uncharacteristic behavior such as cursing and threatening language. This agitated behavior is a result of the impaired person trying to make sense out of a confusing world. Also caregivers may become frightened by this behavior and exhausted by the demands of the impaired loved one.

"How bad is this going to get?" I asked the doctor. He told me that Mom could stay in this stage for a long time. But it will not get any better. The important thing is to be very supportive and not always point out her mistakes. Also, the nurse gave me a list of resources for the elderly and victims of dementia that we used at times.

By the time Mom was diagnosed, Alzheimer's disease was a household word. The first time I heard about this affliction was in the early 1980's when Rita Hayworth was diagnosed. Hayworth had become a movie star with her performance in the 1939 movie *Only Angels Have* Wings.

During her career, she starred in musicals opposite some of the biggest stars such as Fred Astaire, Gene Kelly, and Frank Sinatra. The actress had a sparkling beauty and flawless dancing skills. In Rita Hayworth's career, she appeared in over 60 films and made the cover of *Life* magazine four times. Hayworth's performance in *Gilda* in 1946 made her a superstar. During the 1950s and 1960s, her popularity declined. She made fewer movies and began to drink heavily.

Rita performed in her last feature film, *The Wrath of God* in 1972. In this film, she was having problems with her memory. Her co-star Frank Langella later said that Rita needed cue cards to remember her lines. Also in one scene, a man was off camera prompting her with lines. Rumors spread that her faulty memory was due to alcoholism.

However in 1981, Rita Hayworth was diagnosed with Alzheimer's disease. In hindsight, she suffered from early onset of Alzheimer's disease that was undiagnosed from 1960 when she was only 42 years of age.

At that time, there was not much awareness of the disorder. Hayworth's diagnosis brought the first public attention to this illness. In the following years, her health declined. Her daughter, Princess Yasmin Khan, became her caregiver. Princess Khan became a spokesperson and fundraiser for the Alzheimer's Disease and Related Disorders Association. This organization works to increase public awareness of the disease.

Rita Hayworth died in 1987 at the age of sixty-eight. However, Princess Khan continued her work to bring national attention to this little know disease by establishing the Rita Hayworth Gala, an annual celebrity event that is a most successful fundraiser for Alzheimer's.

Now much attention has been given to this condition since former President Ronald Reagan was diagnosed. Did he know it was going to be his fate? In 1982, the President proclaimed November as "National Alzheimer's Month." Reagan's mother and older brother experienced loss of memory and while in office, the President began joking about his poor memory.

Alzheimer's disease can progress so gradually that in the beginning it is thought of as mild forgetfulness. I wonder how long President Ronald Reagan was running the country with this disease in progress? In his last term, he was bothered by memory lapses, but his mind was well within the realm of normal functioning. What starts out as an absent-minded loss of keys and glasses progresses into moments of total confusion.

By 1992, three years after President Reagan left office, his forgetfulness became very obvious. The former president might be telling a story, and in the middle of it, he would become distracted and forget the conclusion. Reagan was officially diagnosed in 1994. In the beginning of his condition, Reagan still retained his way with words. In an open letter to the American public, Ronald Reagan wrote by hand:

I have recently been told that I am one of the millions of Americans who will be afflicted with Alzheimer's disease. ...Unfortunately as Alzheimer's progresses, the family often bears a heavy burden. I only wish that there were some way I could spare Nancy from this painful experience. ...I now begin the journey that will lead me into the sunset of my life. I know that for America there will always be a bright dawn ahead.[8]

Five months after Ronald Reagan wrote this widely reprinted letter to the American public, the news media reported a conversation between Nancy Reagan and a friend. Mrs. Reagan commented that her husband saw the White House on television but did not remember ever living there.

How could this happen to a powerful figure like Ronald Reagan who lived such a full life? This man was an accomplished actor. Then he went into politics. In 1981, he was elected fortieth President of the United States. A man known as "The Great Communicator" now groped for simple words to use. If a person like Ronald Reagan is suffering from Alzheimer's disease, it could happen to anyone.

I wanted to know more about this disease. What happens to the brain of a person with Alzheimer's? It starts with portions of the brain that become clouded with two separate forms of cellular debris. Clusters of plaque float between the neurons and long black stringy tangles choke the neurons from inside their cell membranes. When the plaques and tangles spread, some neurons lose the ability to transmit messages to one another. The plaques and tangles get so thick that many of the neurons die and the brain begins to shrink.

Since the brain is highly specialized, each clump of neurons affects a specific function such as recalling recent events to recognizing loved ones. This debilitating disease usually progresses slowly over the next five to ten years. It is interesting that when Alzheimer's disease initially attacks a person, the loss of recent memory is what is most apparent. This is because Alzheimer's first attacks the hippocampus which is the area of the brain responsible for short-term memory.

People close to the victim may observe that he or she may be having a little trouble concentrating. However, much of the long-term memory is still intact. The victim may remember incidents from childhood but not remember what he or she had for breakfast. Alzheimer's disease progresses in stages that conform to the development of the human brain in reverse. The last abilities acquired are the first ones forgotten, and the first functions mastered are the last to be taken. The person with Alzheimer's regresses back to birth.

In the beginning stages, a person may become confused

about time and distance. An individual who once was quick with math may have trouble adding a column of numbers. As the impairment progresses, the victim's personality begins to change. An individual who had a great sense of humor may seldom laugh anymore. He or she probably would not even grasp what is amusing about a joke or incident.

As the disease takes over, victims of Alzheimer's could forget their own birthdays, where they live, or the names of close relatives. Eventually, it could rob them of the most basic needs such as being able to feed themselves and taking care of their own elimination process. Alzheimer's is a condition in which degenerative changes occur in the cortex, which is located in the upper level of the brain. It affects the area where thinking, reasoning, and remembering is processed. There is no cure.

7
Why Research Was Held Back

When the German psychiatrist Alois Alzheimer initially identified this destructive brain disorder in 1906, his patient was a woman who died at age fifty-six with severe dementia. After an autopsy was performed, Dr. Alzheimer noted that the brain of this woman showed abnormalities. The damage showed lesions, which harmed the brain cells. Some of these lesions take the form of plaques, patches of dead brain cells. The other abnormality was neurofibrillary tangles, which are twisted threads of protein found within the nerve cells. The plaques and tangles are what destroy the brain cells of Alzheimer's victims. Before the autopsy of this woman in her 50's, the presence of the neurofibrillary tangles had never been described. Therefore, it was this abnormality that was the defining characteristic of a new disease called Alzheimer's.

Unfortunately, the first patient in whom this destructive illness was discovered was so young. Since dementia in people who are sixty-five and younger is quite rare, it led physicians at that time to believe Alzheimer's was a presenile dementia. In the early 1900s, Alzheimer's disease was not considered a major health problem so research was delayed.

In that era, senility was thought to be an inevitable part of aging. If a person lived to be over eighty, society accepted that fate as normal aging. By 1970, it was discovered that dementia is not a natural consequence of the aging process. Also, an important discovery was that younger people with Alzheimer's and older individuals suffering from senility have the same pathological changes in their brains. This discovery suggests that the two dementing illnesses are a single disease.

As we approached the new millennium, a growing interest occurred in researching this devastating illness. There are several reasons for this.

The health conscious "baby boomers" are not accepting brain deterioration as a natural part of growing old, especially since we are approaching that rapidly growing elderly population. Because of the improvements in our living standards, a large portion of our population will live to an advanced age. Alzheimer's disease and other related dementias are not only a threat to those afflicted but to their families and friends.

The financial costs of this disorder may be staggering. The average cost for a person with Alzheimer's disease during a lifetime is $170,000.[9] Seven out of 10 people with this cognitive disorder live at home. Family members provide 75 percent of the caregiving and the remainder is "paid care" which cost the families an average of $12,500 a year.[10] This is beyond what many people could afford so families will eventually seek government subsidy. Therefore, Alzheimer's disease will not only affect the patients and their family and friends, but the financial costs will take an enormous toll on society. The threat of Alzheimer's disease is so great that it is no wonder it has been referred to as "the disease of the century."

With our recent advances in understanding Alzheimer's disease and the realization that this is a major public health issue, we now have a significant increase in research for a cause and treatment of this illness.

8
Antioxidants

Since my mother was in the beginning stages of Alzheimer's disease, I wanted to do everything I could to slow down the deterioration of more brain cells. Was there any way of preventing this from happening? After all, I wondered about my fate. I have always been interested in the benefits of good nutrition and vitamin supplements, so I started to research this area. Researchers have been studying nutritional compounds called antioxidants that are showing promise in the fight against Alzheimer's.

Brain metabolism uses lots of oxygen. This is known as oxidation. However, a side effect of oxidation produces free radicals that are the troublemakers. When cells are attacked by these free radicals, health problems will occur where the cells have been harmed. Research suggests that in Alzheimer's disease, nerve cells are being attacked in the brain by these free radicals.

Antioxidants help deactivate free radicals and help protect cells in the entire body including the brain cells. Our bodies produce a certain amount of antioxidants during normal metabolism. At times, it is just not enough. Research suggests that a diet rich in antioxidants, as well as other nutrients, may be the strongest defense against Alzheimer's. Also, it may be a way of slowing down this disease that is already in progress.

I first asked the physician if I could give Mom and Dad supplemental vitamins and whether any of them would interfere with their medications. He said it would be perfectly safe for them. Along with a multi-vitamin, I gave my parents extra vitamin C and E supplements that are known for their antioxidant properties.

A study was reported in the New England Journal of Medicine in 1997 in which people with Alzheimer's disease were given high doses of vitamin E. It was concluded that the development of symptoms in this controlled group was delayed. Also, this group was reported to have lived longer and was able to stay out of nursing homes longer. They maintained their ability to do everyday tasks longer than the group not given the antioxidants.[11]

Along with the supplements, I tried to always have plenty of fruits and vegetables cut up in the refrigerator so Mom and Dad could have nutritional snacks. They are the best natural source of antioxidants to guard our brain cells against damage from free radicals. Researchers from Tufts University did a study on the fruits and vegetables that best neutralize free radicals. Scientists measure a food's antioxidants in units called oxygen radical absorbency capacities (ORACs). The USDA estimates most people have an intake of 1,200 ORACs daily. Tufts researchers Dr. Ronald Prior and Dr. Guohua Cao are recommending an increase to between 3,000 - 5,000 ORACs units daily to have a significant antioxidant capacity.[12]

At the top of the list for antioxidant potency are blueberries. One cup of blueberries contains 3,200 ORAC units. In the study by Prior and Cao, rats were fed daily doses of blueberry extracts before they were exposed to pure oxygen. The rats that consumed the antioxidant extract had less damage than the group that did not.[13]

Also, some of the other foods reported to have high antioxidant properties are strawberries, raisins, oranges, spinach, beets, peppers, cantaloupe, and watermelon. It is unknown whether vitamin E can prevent Alzheimer's from developing in the first place, but I have been more conscientious about eating these fruits and vegetables. It can't hurt.

Another way to get a healthy dose of antioxidants without worrying about calories is drinking a cup of tea. Researchers at Tufts University found that a 5-ounce cup of black or green tea has 1,246 ORAC units.[14] I am a coffee drinker, but after learning this, I am considering switching to tea.

Red wine is full of antioxidants that come from the skins of grapes. Alcohol is an anti-inflammatory and can boost the good HDL cholesterol and protect the brain from strokes. Medical research is not promoting the excessive use of alcoholic beverages to prevent Alzheimer's disease but acknowledges its antioxidant properties.

There was a study in Bordeaux, France where the alcohol consumed is mostly red wine. The subjects involved a large group of men and women over the age of sixty-five.

The conclusion of this research showed a possible link between the consumption of red wine and a lower risk of Alzheimer's.

Another study headed by Dr. Egemen Savaskan of the University of Basel in Switzerland researched the effects of red wine. This study suggests that a molecule called resveratrol that is found in red wine may protect the brain cells against Alzheimer's by mopping up free radicals that attack the brain.[15]

An important factor in these studies is drinking in moderation. There is no healthy benefit in excessive drinking. Consuming large quantities of alcohol can kill cells and cause brain atrophy along with the destruction of other organs in the body. If you do not want to consume a glass of red wine on a daily basis, you could drink purple grape juice. This is full of antioxidants without the alcohol.

Great news for chocolate lovers! Chocolate is derived from the beans of the cacao tree and is brimming with antioxidants. Chocolate contains polyphenols which are the same class of antioxidants found in fruits and vegetables. According to the data from United States Department of Agriculture, dark chocolate per 100 grams has twice the ORAC of milk chocolate.[16]

We are exposed to constant assaults by free radical chemicals that turn our bodies and brains rancid. It makes sense to fight against those attacks. One of the most important steps you could take to save your brain from gradual deterioration is to eat a diet rich in antioxidants. Why wait until eighty? Let's start now. More importantly, let's teach our children good nutritional habits.

Doesn't an antioxidant boost sound good for that afternoon droop? A cup of tea or cocoa with a slice of my homemade blueberry pie. Here is my recipe made from scratch.

2 cups flour	1½ pints of fresh blueberries
¼ tsp. baking powder	
1 tablespoon granulated sugar	½ cup granulated sugar
1 tablespoon brown sugar	¼ cup brown sugar
1 stick of butter (softened)	1 teaspoon cinnamon
2 egg yolks	½ cup chopped walnuts
1 cup sour cream	
1 tablespoon brown sugar	

For the crust, combine first four ingredients in a mixing bowl. Break butter into flour mixture. Crumble with hands until flour looks like cornmeal. Put in an ungreased pie dish. Pat evenly going up the sides of dish. Place fresh blueberries over pastry. Combine sugars, cinnamon, and walnuts. Sprinkle over blueberries. Bake for 15 minutes at 350 degrees. While baking, combine egg yolks, sour cream, and brown sugar. Then pour the mixture over blueberries and bake for 30 minutes longer. The pie tastes best when made a day ahead for everything to mold together. Enjoy.

In my quest for finding ways to reduce the risks of Alzheimer's disease, I stock my cabinets with spices that might be potent fighters against dementia. One common spice is curry powder that has a compound in its principal ingredient, turmeric.

Sally Frautschy, Ph.D., of University of California at Los Angeles did a study on what role curcumin might have. She fed a diet rich in curcumin to mice that had been genetically programmed to develop Alzheimer's disease. The animals showed the inflammation of neurological tissue was reduced. Also, the plaque was clear between the nerve cells. After consuming this spicy diet of curcumin, the mice were better able to handle the maze. Dr. Frautschy's study showed that there were changes in the brains of the mice that were responsible for the improvement in their memories.

This spice is used as a food preservative and herbal medicine in India. Alzheimer's disease in India with patients between 70 and 79 years of age is 4.4-fold less than in the United States.[17]

Adding curry powder while preparing dinner may not only perk up your meal, but it may be able to enhance brain activity as well. There are other brain-friendly spices that I keep on hand. Rosemary and ginger contain compounds similar to curcumin. This should produce the same effects.

While cooking, I think of the spices that I am adding as an internal suit of armor to repel or neutralize the chemical attacks on my body and brain. Some of my favorite antioxidants to use for flavor while preparing dinner are onions and parsley. One cup of chopped onion has 720 ORAC units, and parsley has been known to stimulate brain activity. And for my all time favorite, garlic. Lots of it!

Garlic has long been known for its medicinal properties to ward away germs. But I am excited to learn it has powerful antioxidant properties. One clove contains 1,939 ORAC units. I love a good pork roast simmering with garlic, onions, rosemary, and parsley served with roasted red peppers. If you are serving this to that special someone in your life and think the evening may lead to some serious kissing, top the meal off with some fresh mint.

In 1986, David Snowdon, Ph.D. of the University of Kentucky where he is a Professor of Neurology started the Nun Study which is an ongoing research project examining 678 Sisters of Notre Dame religious congregation ranging in age from 75 to 106. Dr. Snowdon found two other nutrients that may also be important: lycopene and folate. He found lycopene to be associated with longevity more than any other nutrient in his study.

Also, this nutrient seems to be extremely protective against mental impairment as we age. In Dr. Snowdon's findings, a group of the nuns in this study were tested for levels of lycopene in their blood. Those found with the highest levels of this antioxidant in their blood were more self-reliant with daily activities such as walking, dressing, bathing, and feeding themselves[18]

Lycopene is a powerful antioxidant with a reddish color. Some of the best sources of this potent antioxidant are tomato paste, tomato ketchup, tomato sauce, tomato soup, and watermelon. Learning about this study of lycopene was good news for me. I will no longer feel guilty about eating that extra slice of pizza. It may not be good for my waistline, but after all, I am protecting my brain.

Folate or folic acid is the other nutrient in this study. Dr. Snowdon found a definite link between low levels of folate in the blood and increased risks of brain atrophy. In his research involving thirty nuns, the results were that the sisters with the lowest levels of folic acid in their blood had the most massive deterioration of the brain."[19]

Folate works in conjunction with vitamin B_{12} in breaking down the compound homocysteine. Scientists have found that homocysteine contributes to the buildup of plaque in the arteries that could interfere with the blood flow to the brain. This process could play a role in the development of Alzheimer's. The best sources of folate are from leafy green vegetables, dried beans, citrus fruits, and nuts. Most experts agree that the amount of folic acid needed to protect the brain against Alzheimer's is 400 micrograms. This amount is found in most multiple vitamin tablets.

Coenzyme Q10 is another antioxidant that scientists are now concentrating on to rejuvenate the brain. For years, researchers studied CoQ10 in heart cells. Their findings showed a lack of CoQ10 slowed the heart's energy. This contributed to heart failure. When levels of this antioxidant were restored, it reenergized the heart function.

Now scientists are turning their attention to CoQ10 and its relationship to the brain. It is known that CoQ10 levels decline as we age. Some researchers feel that adding the supplement to our diet will help protect our brain from normal aging.

One of the culprits in depleting our supply of CoQ10 is cholesterol-lowering drugs. Statins may be necessary to clean our arteries, but if you need to take them, it may be a good idea to replenish the brain with the antioxidant supplement CoQ10.

Another antioxidant is ginkgo biloba, which is a nonprescription drug to revive failing memory. Ginkgo increases circulation of blood and oxygen to the capillaries of the brain. Ginkgo is said to be helpful in restoring mild mental deficiency in concentration and confusion that comes from normal aging. Ginkgo has been approved in Germany for a decade for this condition.

9
Exercise

Since 1990, researchers have been investigating possible lifestyle links to Alzheimer's disease. They have found some interesting connections. It is not only our dietary habits. How we exercise, handle stress and manage our emotions can affect the health of our brain and may influence our chance of developing Alzheimer's. This condition seems to develop slowly due to many factors and a breakdown of the body's different systems. A common sense approach to reduce the chances of this illness is to keep each system functioning as well as possible.

Many of the healthy lifestyle tips to protect our brain could also be used in protecting our heart. In Dr. Snowdon's study, he found physical exercise an important factor in preventing or delaying dementia. Exercise improves blood flow nourishing the brain cells with oxygen and nutrients. It has been known for years that exercise is important to maintain a healthy heart. It helps prevent strokes, diabetes, high blood pressure, and high cholesterol. All of these illnesses can increase the chances of Alzheimer's. Dr. Snowdon's suggestion for the single most important thing we should do as we age is walk.[20]

Other studies have been done on how physical exercise benefits the brain. Robert P. Friedland, M.D., a professor of neurology at Case Western Reserve University School of Medicine was the lead author in the study reported in the *Proceedings of National Academy of Science*. In this research Dr. Friedman concluded that people with higher levels of activity were about three and a half times **less** likely to get Alzheimer's disease than those with lower levels.[21]

Researchers are finding that consistency is more important than intensity of the workout. How much exercise is needed to preserve our memory? Most major health organizations such as the American College of Sports Medicine, the National Institutes of Health, and the American Heart Association agree that about 30 minutes a day of moderate activity is all we need. This could be done as walking, swimming, participating in sports, gardening or just doing chores around the house. If you find an exercise that you really enjoy, you are more likely to make it a life long practice. To incorporate more exercise in my daily routine, I make it a point to take the stairs instead of elevators and escalators.

10
High Blood Pressure and Cholesterol

Another area that doctors have suspected increases the risk of Alzheimer's is high blood pressure and high cholesterol. Recently, a study of over 1,400 people was completed and reported in the *British Medical Journal* in June 2001. This group of people had either high blood pressure or high cholesterol in their 40s and 50s and did **not** do anything about it over the next 21 years. This group increased their risks of developing Alzheimer's over 200 percent. People with high blood pressure were 2.3 times more likely to develop Alzheimer's. The high cholesterol group was 2.1 times more prone. People with both conditions are at risk at 3.5 times above normal.[22]

Steve Seiner, M.D., an instructor of psychiatry at Harvard Medical School, feels that this study supports the idea of taking care of our bodies and our basic health when we're younger in order to help lower our risk for Alzheimer's disease later in life.[23]

Rudolph Tanzi, Ph.D., professor of neurology at Harvard Medical School and the author of *Decoding Darkness: The Search for Genetic Causes of Alzheimer's Disease*, feels there is a strong possibility that high cholesterol levels may add to a production of protein formation that plays a key role in accumulating plaque in the brain. Dr. Tanzi says, "We're seeing more and more that what's bad for the heart is bad for the brain. With any risk factor linked to heart disease, you need to pay attention to it for Alzheimer's as well."[24] This content has been reproduced with the permission of HealthAtoZ (www.healthatoz.com).

Statins such as Lipitor, Zocor, and Pravachol are used daily throughout the world to lower cholesterol which reduces heart attacks and strokes. Recent findings suggest that statins guard against mental decline as well. Dr. Benjamin Wolozin of Loyola University Medical Center said, "What we found was that patients taking statins have a 60 to 73 percent reduction in the risk of Alzheimer's disease."[25]

11
Increase Risk from Depression

People who have had a history of chronic depression may be at an increased risk of developing Alzheimer's. From Dr. Snowdon's research and his own study, he concludes that a history of depression can increase the chances of developing Alzheimer's. Scientists found that chronic depression can cause shrinkage of the hippocampus, which is the memory center of the brain. This shrinkage is similar to what is seen in Alzheimer's.[26]

If depression could increase our risks, I wonder if laughter and joy in life could help guard us against Alzheimer's. Dr. Snowdon is still in the process of researching this area. However, his data found that a positive attitude can help fight against disease in general. In his study with the nuns, Dr. Snowdon and his team were able to find a definite connection between a positive attitude and longevity. The nuns who had a positive outlook on life showed a survival increase of 6.9 years.[27]

12
Guard Against Head Injuries

Researchers say that the third leading cause of Alzheimer's disease behind age and genetics is a history of head injury. This is commonly seen in boxers who endured repeated blows to the head. Dr. Tanzi is concerned about children using their heads to strike a soccer ball. In soccer, this technique is called heading. Tanzi warns parents to be aware of the risks before allowing their children to use their head to hit a soccer ball.

"If you really want to be safe, don't let them do it. It's not worth risking the rest of their lives," Tanzi warns. "Common sense would argue that heading a heavy object coming in at a fast speed causes head trauma and head trauma is a risk factor for Alzheimer's."[28] This content has been reproduced with the permission of HealthAtoZ (www.healthatoz.com).

There are a series of compelling studies from the University of Pennsylvania School of Medicine that demonstrate a link between trauma of the brain and Alzheimer's disease. In this study, scientists concluded that shortly after brain trauma, a plaque forms in the brain similar to that of an Alzheimer's victim.

Researchers stressed the importance of protecting our heads from trauma. It is even more important to safeguard our children, especially during the early years when injuries have an even longer period of time to gestate into plaque buildup, which could become a problem.[29] Parents need to be conscientious about seeing that their children wear helmets when riding a bike or rollerblading.

13
Use It or Lose It

What happens when we push our brains to learn by reading and achieving higher education? Some studies suggest that we build up a cognitive reserve that may help us avoid noticeable effects of brain damage. Cognitive reserve is thought to be a measure of brain capacity. "The theory is that cognitive reserve—greater levels of which might be marked by educational achievement—may act as a cushion against intellectual impairment," said Margaret Gatz Ph.D., a professor of psychology at the University of Southern California, Los Angeles. Dr. Gatz, the lead researcher in this study, found evidence of the phenomenon by studying twins. The results of this study show when data is analyzed for the overall population, low education is a significant factor for Alzheimer's and other forms of dementia.[30]

However, the most dramatic evidence in the theory to "use it or lose it" comes from a study that was reported in the *Proceedings of National Academy of Sciences.* This study showed how people had spent their leisure time when they were in their early adulthood and middle age. Researchers found that individuals whose leisure time centered around mentally stimulating activities such as reading, writing, crossword puzzles, chess, or a musical instrument were two and a half times **less** likely to develop Alzheimer's later in life than people who enjoyed more passive activities such as watching television or talking on the phone.[31]

The study's lead author Robert P. Friedland, M.D., a professor of neurology at Case Western Reserve University School of Medicine remarked, "Intellectual stimulation in early and middle adulthood did not provide absolute protection against Alzheimer's in late adulthood, but the activities could delay the disease for years."[32]

Dr. Richard Whiting, a geriatrician at Sunshine Hospital agrees with the research. "The development of a stronger neuronal network makes the brain more resistant to early onset of Alzheimer's. This research sends an important message to young adults that their actions now have great bearings on future physical and mental health."

After reading about these studies, I need to be more aware of exercising my mental capacities. Like most people, I have gotten into the habit of allowing modern technology do some very basic work. I decided to give up my pocket calculator and add the numbers in my head. Also, I need to turn off the television and pick up a book more often.

The prudent middle-aged adults are concerned about building their nest egg for retirement. In addition to keeping abreast of 401K and stocks, the baby boomers need to build "cognitive reserve" accounts to draw on for those golden years. It may be a good idea to follow the same theory with our brains as we would for our finances.

Since the early 1990's, researchers have been studying Alzheimer's disease and how it is associated with lifestyles. They have found some interesting connections. Evidence suggests that the strategies for healthy living and aging may help to reduce the risks of Alzheimer's disease. These tactics include a balanced diet with plenty of fruits and vegetables, controlling blood pressure and cholesterol, exercising your mind and body, guarding against head injuries and staying socially active. It's never too early or late to start.

14
Going with the Flow

The following months were a tremendous growing experience for me. It helped to think of my caregiving as an education. When I started thinking of the daily problems as an inevitable part of life and viewed them as a potential teacher, I felt a weight lifted off my shoulders. Instead of resisting and struggling, I embraced the situation and learned a great deal about coping skills. I realized I had to help Mom but could not keep fighting her for everything. It was too exhausting. However, I actually was proud of myself for thinking of creative ways to deal with the disease.

I looked at Mom with her uncombed hair. The last time I tried to comb her hair, we got into a terrible fight. It had to be done, but so much time and energy would be wasted on arguing.

One of the first things I learned that was helpful in coping with Mom was to breathe before speaking. When I would take a deep breath, I had much better results. This strategy is quite simple. It involves nothing more than pausing and breathing. The tension and agitation would leave me, and my voice sounded much softer. Also, I looked at the situation with added perspective and increased patience. This tranquil feeling actually became contagious. When I spoke calmly, Mom seemed more compliant.

"Mom, I wonder if you could help me," I said.

"Yeah, what?" she asked.

"You know, Mom," I began, "a lot of my friends have been telling me that I can do hair really well. So I was thinking that I should go into business and do hair for people. I think I could make a lot of money."

"That's a good idea. You should do it," she agreed.

"Well before I start charging people, I may need a little more practice. Would you mind if I practiced washing and setting your hair?" I asked.

"Sure, you could practice on my hair," she said pleasantly.

That was easy. Mom still wanted to feel needed. So as long as she was helping me, instead of me helping her, it was perfectly all right. I learned that a person with this debilitating disease must be treated with dignity. I washed and set Mom's hair that day and then combed it. We both stared in the mirror admiring this work of art. Mom looked pretty with her nice hairdo and pleasant look on her face.

"Well, I better get going, Mom. I still have a lot to do in my own house." Then I noticed the sweater she was wearing had some spots on it. Now how am I going to get that sweater off her so I could wash it?

"Mom, I might be going out tonight, but I don't have anything to wear. I was wondering if I could borrow your sweater?" I asked.

"Okay," she said.

"Thanks," I said. "Come on, let's find another top for you to wear."

We got another one from her drawer. She put it on and looked especially nice.

"I'll bring your sweater back tomorrow," I said.

"Oh Honey, you don't have to rush with it," she said.

We parted that day with a warm, loving feeling between us.

I don't know if this is lying, manipulating, or just using common sense, but I had to learn to be a master at it.

The first step in meeting this challenge was accepting that this was a disease. Our mother-daughter relationship had to change. I could no longer reason with Mom but still had to treat her with dignity. Everyone's life is a journey of discovery. As I gained more patience and understanding, I was able to cope better. There were still frustrating days, but I tried to handle the problems that arose daily as more of a dance and less of a battle. I used the philosophy of going with the flow, which was the beginning of finding inner peace.

15
Taking Precautions

Things continued the same for a while. I tried to assist Mom without making it obvious. She still attempted to do things like cooking until a small fire started in the kitchen. Luckily, the alarm went off which is connected to the fire company. That is one of the nice features of living in the apartment building for senior citizens. The police and firefighters arrived. The building had to be evacuated. No one was hurt but Mom was terribly upset. I never did find out any details about the fire. Mom looked disturbed for the next few days, but she could not remember why.

We realized that Mom definitely should not be using the stove. At this point, Dad was still driving so we decided that the two of them should go out for meals. This would then eliminate grocery shopping, cooking, and washing dishes. I made an attempt to convince Mom that everybody goes out to eat these days.

"Mom, after all the years you cooked, you deserve a break," I said. "And besides, Dad likes to go out for dinner now. You get to enjoy each other and there's no work."

"Well all right," she said hesitantly.

"Why bother cooking," I said.

"I guess nobody cooks anymore," she agreed.

That was settled. However, just in case Mom had any ideas of heating something up on the stove, I took away the pots and pans.

The caregiver must protect the memory-impaired person from what he or she cannot do. However, it is impossible to force a person suffering from Alzheimer's into our idea of reality. Emphasizing an individual's limitations only lowers his or her self-esteem. Try to avoid confrontation and conflict with a person who is cognitively impaired. Focus on the remaining strengths of the victim. This is quite a challenge for the caregivers who are desperately trying to protect their loved ones.

16
Make Allowance for Change of Plans

One of the big lessons I learned with being a caregiver is I had to take time for myself. I continued to make plans. Dom and I had our pizza date at Palermo's every Friday night. We still went out with our friends. Our friends knew our situation so I would tell them when making plans that if an emergency should occur with my parents, we will have to cancel. But I made them assure me that they would still participate in whatever social we planned. That took a lot of pressure off me, especially if we were buying tickets to an event. Without that agreement with my friends, I probably would not make plans.

There were several times that I came late to a social event and sometime plans had to be postponed or completely canceled. At first, I was very disappointed and sometimes angry. But gradually, it became helpful to expect that a certain percentage of plans will change or be interrupted. If allowances are made in my mind for the inevitable, I am able to chalk it up to one of life's happenings. Life goes on. Changing plans became another learning experience in going with the flow.

17
The Accident

In January 1999, Dom had a business trip in Atlanta, and he wanted me to accompany him. Thank God I had Aunt Anna. My aunt was Mom's younger sister. She was a big help during this time. My aunt is a super conscientious person so I felt very comfortable leaving for a few days. I remember having a very pleasant time in Atlanta. While Dom went to conferences in the day, I shopped and swam in the hotel pool. In the evening, we were able to have dinner together. It was really great getting away and so important. The long weekend went by quickly, and we were back home. Aunt Anna reported that everything went well with no major catastrophes. The only thing Aunt Anna said was Mom kept asking over and over again when was I coming back? Why did I have to go? Well, now I feel refreshed and ready to get back to the routine.

One of Mom's favorite things to do is enjoy nature while walking. Going for walks has always been part of the day's activities, and she was still so physically fit. So the day after I got back from my trip, I rushed over to Mom's so we could go for a long walk. It was a little brisk out so I mentioned to Mom she needed a hat.

She never liked wearing hats so she said, "I don't need a hat. It's not cold outside."

By this time, I knew not to get into an argument with her so I said, "Well, I'm wearing a hat. Why don't we just bring one for you? You could put it on if you get cold?"

Mom agreed on that and as soon as we went out the door, she put on her hat. That morning we had a lovely walk while I told her about my trip. I did not have to do too much of her housework or wash because Aunt Anna had done it all. So this was quite pleasant. After about an hour of walking, we started to go back inside.

THAT'S WHEN IT HAPPENED!

Mom tripped on one little step going into the building and fell. She tried to get up but couldn't. There were people outside so someone ran to call an ambulance while I stayed with Mom. While she was on the ground, I remember being glad Mom had her hat. When the ambulance arrived, the paramedics lifted her onto the stretcher, and I got into the ambulance with her. On the way to the hospital, I felt as if this was unreal. Maybe this is the reason I get through these disasters with complete self-control. I feel that I am watching a movie.

Mom was taken into the emergency room and given x-rays. And we waited. The result of this fall was a broken hip and shoulder. Walking—the one activity Mom loved so much will now have to be stopped. The next day Mom had to undergo surgery for a hip replacement. I had been calm and in control up to the point that Mom was being wheeled away on the gurney. Then I was overcome with emotion and fright of the unknown.

"Please God, don't let my mother suffer," I said to myself.

It seemed like an eternity that I waited for the doctor. As I sat in the waiting room, I relived the accident. I should have stayed in Atlanta a couple more days. Why did we have to go for a walk? I went over and over the events in my mind to see if there was any way this could have been prevented.

Mom always walked so fast. I remember opening the door to the building when she tripped on that step. She must have climbed that step thousands of times. I should have been holding on to her.

"OH DAMN IT!" She was always so agile and coordinated all her life. She had the athletic body and ability that I wanted but did not inherit. Why didn't I realize that she could have forgotten that little step? Or why didn't I realize that her coordination could have slightly declined with Alzheimer's?

18
Dealing with Guilt

I was being weighed down by this feeling of guilt. My energy was depleting from the extra emotional baggage. I knew that I was going to need my stamina to help Mom. So I had to cut myself some slack. In doing so, I gained a clearer perspective. How could I possibly know Mom was going to trip? This is a setback, but I have to get back on track.

First I have to eliminate all thoughts of what I should or could have done differently to prevent Mom from falling. This kind of thinking serves no purpose. I needed to use all my energy productively. Life is what it is and no amount of condemning myself for being unable to predict Mom's fall would change anything. Learning to dismiss these negative thoughts was another step in my growing experience. I tried thinking of this mishap as another learning opportunity. Also, I know that I am doing the best I can. I will expect setbacks and when they occur, I must stay loving toward myself because I am human.

When the doctor came out, he said the surgery went well, however, Mom would have to get therapy in rehab. With the hip surgery, the nurses had to get her up and moving quickly. I remember sitting in her room with Dad the next day. The nurses very cautiously got her out of bed and held her up for a few minutes. Dad and I looked at each other, and I remember the shocked look on his face. He couldn't believe this was happening. He just shook his head in disbelief.

While I was witnessing this scene, a picture came into my mind. It was a day a couple years ago. Mom and I went to the library in Norristown. There is this long flight of steps you must climb to get inside. By the time we reached the top, I was out of breath. Mom walked right up without any problem. She even seemed annoyed with me that I was too slow. That had always been a problem. All of her life, Mom moved faster than most people.

"Can't you move any faster," she would say. In that way, she was incompatible with the rest of us.

Her life long friend Betty said, "I always picture Fran when she worked at the pants factory in Bridgeport. She walked over that bridge everyday to and from work. Fran always moved like lightning."

Whether it was walking, cleaning, shoveling snow, or answering the telephone, Mom had to do it quickly. She also said it was easier for her to do things herself than to wait to get it done. It did become quite comfortable for all of us to let her do the work at her fast speed. But as I watched these nurses hold her up, I muffled my cry, "Mommy."

After a week in the hospital, Mom had to go to a rehab. She would have to learn to walk and regain use of her arm. Mom was very frightened and confused by this whole episode. With the anesthesia, drugs, and unfamiliar surroundings, her mental state made a very noticeable decline. In addition to this, she was very uncooperative. She did not want to go to rehab. She was in terrible pain and did not know why all these strange people were forcing her to walk. Many times she just refused to go. That became so frustrating for me because I knew that if she did not get therapy for her hip, she might never be able to walk again. So I had to be at the rehab whenever she was scheduled for therapy to insist that she go.

I tried to give her confidence by going with her so she would not be afraid of all the strangers. It was torture for both of us. In addition to being in pain and afraid, she seemed to lose her appetite which was making her very weak. I did not feel that she was going to live through this.

After about three weeks in this rehab, her insurance no longer covered the payments. They said she has made all the progress she is going to by being there. There was no way she would be able to go back to her apartment with Dad. She needed someone now to help her physically as well as mentally. Just getting dressed and in and out of bed was going to be a chore. She would have to go into a nursing home. Now, Mom needed 24-hour care.

I immediately started visiting the local nursing homes. It was so odd. I never pictured my mother like these old people. They were the living dead. Now my parents were responsible for paying for nursing care. Another thought ran through my mind, and it came with a bitter feeling. Mom and Dad lived so frugally all their lives. They were a product of the Depression but never seemed to grow with the times. Instead of enjoying vacations and many of the pleasures of life, they now will use their savings for a nursing home.

19
Life Isn't Fair

Mom would be released from the rehab in three days. She was able to walk and get out of bed with help. She needed someone to bathe and dress her. She was also very confused and afraid of all these strange people and surroundings. She had no appetite and had lost about twenty pounds. I knew that the nursing home was going to confuse and frighten her even more. Why did my mother have to suffer like this? She never had an easy life. She was not the type of person who talked about her misfortunes, but once in a while she would open up to me.

I started thinking about Mom as a child being so poor and not having medical attention. When she was a baby, she had a high fever that caused her eye to weaken. With one weak eye, she would unconsciously use her strong one. After a couple years of only using one eye, Mom lost all sight out of her left eye. Then, this caused the eye to roll uncontrollably. My heart ached when I thought of her being afraid to go to school because kids made fun of her. Picturing her running home because some mean boys were calling her names and throwing stones at her made me fill up with tears. How could anyone be so cruel to my mother? Maybe that's why Mom always had the habit of moving so fast.

In the past when tragedy occurred, it has been easy for me to slump into a depression. I start thinking of every tragedy that our family endured and relive it. Then all these feelings bombarded me. There was the devastation of finding out that Chuckie was born with Down Syndrome in an era that society had very little knowledge about this condition. Our family had to deal with it without the resources and support groups that they have today. Most of that burden fell on Mom, but it certainly changed the course of all of our lives. I thought of other injustices that our family went through, and I was getting angrier and more depressed. Why did my life have to be interrupted with this?

"LIFE ISN'T FAIR!" I thought.

For the next couple days, I spent a lot of time wallowing and complaining about what's wrong with life. I was heartbroken to see Mom in such anguish. If only it was just a physical problem. She would be able to help herself in addition to me helping her. But it was physical and mental. I argued with myself.

Maybe she could come and live with me. I will probably be at the nursing home every day anyway. But if Mom stays with me, I will have no life at all. I will not even be able to go to the grocery store and be comfortable leaving her. She might try to get up and fall. What about my job? I had been at Colonial School District for fourteen years. I had a good job as a Theme Reader and enjoyed it. But it only was part time. I don't know what to do. I did have room in the house. Kris was away at school so her bedroom was available. What about Dom? Is it fair to ask him to make this sacrifice? If I had to care for my mother at our house for 24 hours a day, we couldn't have much of a marriage. What am I going to do?

I was still confused when I went to the grocery store the next day. I was in my own world as I automatically pushed the cart up and down the aisles getting my groceries. As I was reaching for my box of Cheerios, I noticed a familiar face. It was my friend Marge. I was somewhat embarrassed to see her. I heard a rumor that she was not well. I knew that she was on some medical leave from her job, but I really did not know what was wrong.

"Marge, how are you?" I asked. We started talking in the cereal aisle.

At first it was a little awkward, but then she started to open up to me. She told me she had cancer. I wasn't too surprised because I assumed it was something very serious. Marge told me she was facing a rough road ahead of her. She was trying to stay positive and was determined to do everything possible to win this fight for her life. Marge was only in her forties. I am not used to hearing sickness like this among my peers. Again I thought, **"LIFE IS UNFAIR."**

I left the market somewhat uncomfortable about this situation. Our conversation kept coming in and out of my mind all day along with my own problems. I felt so bad for my friend. Her future looked grim with operations and chemotherapy. At her age, life should not be doctors and hospitals. It made me feel very lucky that I was so healthy.

I heard once that people come into your life for a reason. Maybe it was no accident that I met Marge at the market. That day I made a decision. I wanted to take Mom home.

I started to formulate a plan. When Dom came home, I discussed it with him. He said, "You know how hard it is going to be for you. You won't even be able to leave the house." I told him of my plan. I would hire help with the money that was going to go to the nursing home, and Dad could come over to sit with Mom every day so I could get my errands done. If it becomes an impossible situation, we would then resort to placing her in a facility. For my own peace of mind, I have to try. So it was decided. Instead of going to the nursing home, Mom would come to my house.

I really feel that meeting Marge in the market that day was the deciding factor. Also seeing her determination and courage, gave me a better perspective on life and its injustices.

Life is not fair and maybe it was never intended to be fair. I needed to recognize that fact. I mistakenly thought that since we have been through our share of misfortunes, we are now owed a great life.

Changing my outlook on life required hard work. I had to learn to redirect my internal dialogue. Instead of making maladaptive statements such as "This is terrible," or "I can't stand it," I would practice more adaptive statements such as "I don't like this, but I can handle it." Or "this is unfortunate but not terrible." I even went as far as writing these adaptive messages to myself and placing them on the refrigerator and bathroom mirror. I would read these notes often, and they would serve as a reminder to me that I could cope with the situation.

Once I made peace with the fact that life is not fair, I stopped feeling angry at the situation. Well, it's not "life's job" to make everything perfect. It is our challenge to adjust. With this new insight, I am reminded that everyone is dealt a different hand, and I started learning to use adversity to bring out strength that I did not know I had. Now a change occurred, and I had to meet the challenge.

20
Meeting the Challenge

Mom's insurance covered help to come to the house for about three weeks. A physical therapist came to help her walk and strengthen her arm. An aid came to assist in bathing and dressing her. Mom still did not have much of an appetite and was wasting away. Then it hit me. Maybe the antidepressant that was prescribed caused her appetite to be suppressed. I asked the doctor about that and he said it could very well be. A different antidepressant was prescribed. Immediately Mom's appetite came back, and she gradually regained her weight and strength. She also seemed much calmer being around familiar people, and her mental state was better. She continued to do her hip and shoulder exercises with the therapist coming to the house but did not understand why she had to go through this procedure everyday. Mom had no recollection of falling or being in the hospital and rehab.

Miraculously, my mother walked again without as much as a limp. I attribute this to being in such great physical condition all of her life. Her shoulder gradually healed, but it never came back 100 percent.

Life was less hectic with Mom living at my house. I didn't have to keep running to the hospital and did not have to contend with begging her to go to rehab. She did much better with her therapy in the familiar surroundings.

With Mom's physical state back to normal, it was much easier to take care of her. I still was able to maintain my job and social life. I just had to be content that things were not going to be the same and had to be willing to adjust my life. When the insurance would no longer pay for an aid, I helped Mom with her shower and hair in the day when nobody else was home using the bathroom.

Several appliances made showering easier and the bathroom much safer. A raised toilet seat is easier for an impaired person to maneuver. A padded seat is comfortable when an individual must sit for an extended period of time. This is also essential for many elderly people who develop pressure sores. Also grab bars will help your loved one get on and off the toilet. For showering, it is much safer sitting on a bath seat. Also, a hand held hose reduces the bath time crisis. The seat is safer and the controlled flow of water is less upsetting. Also, a bathmat that does not slip is essential on the floor, and a rubber mat is needed for the bottom of the tub.

I learned to first assemble everything needed so I would not have to leave Mom alone in the bathtub. Two towels, washcloths, baby powder, body lotion, and a bathrobe.

Mom was able to wash herself although she had to be reminded one step at a time to wash each area. Before rinsing the soap off in the shower, I made sure she tested the water temperature first. Then I used two big towels to dry her. I put powder in any creases and folds in the skin and lotion on the dry areas of the skin.

Many elderly people are prone to sores and rashes, which could cause infections so I always looked for those signs. Also, it is important to pay attention to an elderly person's feet. Corns, calluses, and bunions can be quite painful. Toenails need to be trimmed regularly so they do not curl back against the toe. Mom had a recurring corn growing on the small toe. I used over-the counter corn medication and padding which made it more comfortable to walk.

Then we went into the bedroom where her clothes were laid out for the day. Everything is washable. Slacks with elastic waistbands and slip on tops. One tip I learned was to spray her tops with Scotch Gard repellent. If she spilled something on them, it would not stain. Loose fitting clothing is much more practical. Short cotton socks and sneakers with Velcro. Avoid slippers or shoes with slick soles that slide on rugs. This could prevent a disaster.

Then I would supervise Mom with her oral hygiene. Mom was able to brush her own teeth. I just had to remind her. After brushing, she rinsed with a pleasing mouthwash. The first time I gave Mom the mouthwash, she swallowed it. After that, I reminded her to swish the liquid around her mouth and then spit it out. It helped to demonstrate this right before she took the glass.

Mom always wore make-up, so I would dust her face with light facial powder and add blush to her cheeks for some color. I chose a pastel lipstick. Mascara and eye shadow were not necessary and would get too involved. Mom always took pride in the way she looked so when her hygiene and grooming were finished, I encouraged her to look in the mirror to see how nice she looked. This did wonders for her morale.

Dental checkups are important for the impaired person. Even mildly forgetful people neglect their teeth. This puts them at risk of developing oral infections. Also, poor teeth or loose fitting dentures could lead to pain and poor nutrition which will increase mental confusion. The caregiver may not detect cavities, sores, and abscesses so it is important to find a dentist who is compassionate and understanding when working on a person with Alzheimer's. When Mom had her dental checkup, I would stay in the examining room talking to her and putting her at ease while Dr. Berger worked on her teeth.

When I did my errands, Mom would come with me. She

liked going out, and it was great for her mental state. She would be with me at the market, hairdresser, and mall. When we went to Sal's Hairstylist, Mom got her hair done along with me. She had her own hairdresser, Rosie, who cut her hair in a short, attractive style that was easy for me to wash and comb. While Mom was sitting under the hairdryer, I gave her a glass of water. This is important if a person is susceptible to dehydration. Also, it is important to keep checking the temperature on the hairdryer.

Dad would stay with her the days I went to work. Since my job was close to home, I would come back at lunchtime to check on things.

By May of 1999, my mother recovered well physically. Mentally she was back to where she was before her fall. There may have been a slight decline, but it was not too noticeable. Maybe she wasn't making any major mistakes because I was doing everything for her. She could still have a reasonable conversation. She still worried about Chuckie.

Once a week, Dad would pick up Chuckie and take him to visit Mom. We still went to her apartment often. I had to clean there and pick up Dad's wash. She would come with me and remember that it was her apartment. She kept saying that she wanted to stay in her own place.

By the end of May, Mom was adamant that she wanted to be in her own apartment, and I felt she was ready. So we started the routine again. I would come every day to help my parents, and they would go out for their meals. I packed away all knickknacks and unnecessary furniture. Simplifying life is the key. Also, I got rid of throw rugs. They could be hazardous. So we got into a routine that worked, and it went fairly well. Once in a while, there would be a drastic lapse in Mom's memory.

21
Dealing with Memory Lapses

One day I went in Mom's apartment, and she looked distraught. "Mom, what is the matter?" I asked.

"I CAN'T FIND THE BABY!" she cried.

"What baby?" I asked.

"YOU KNOW! THE BABY!"

"Mom, there are no babies here. I use to be your baby. Then you had Chuckie, but we grew up. Remember?"

Mom looked perplexed.

I continued, "You baby-sat for Denise and Krissy once in awhile, but they grew up. So there are no more babies." The look of fear left her face and was replaced with relief.

"It has been a long time since you had a baby," I said. "You must have been dreaming."

"Oh yeah, I guess you're right. But I got scared for a minute," she said. I tried to brush it off quickly and not make her dwell on these mistakes.

Another time when I walked in, Mom was shaking.

"I DON'T KNOW WHERE MY MOTHER IS!" she cried.

I looked at Mom and saw a frightened little girl. My heart was breaking for her now. What should I say? Do I lie and say her mother will be back soon or tell her the truth? My gut feeling was to be gentle but truthful. I sat down and put my arm around her. "Mom, don't you remember that your mother died a long time ago," I said.

"MY MOTHER IS DEAD!" she gasped.

"Mom," I said gently, "your mother lived a long life. But she died about 30 years ago."

Mom thought for a long time with a bewildered look on her face.

"Well—I—sort of remember now. But—it seems like she was just here," she said.

Now the confused look turned to sadness. Mom was feeling the sorrow of losing her mother.

"Mom," I said, "maybe it seems that way because your mother loves you so much and is your guardian angel. She is right here on your shoulder watching over you and will never leave you. So you have your mother protecting you. And you have me right here taking care of you."

She seemed comforted with that explanation. I remember holding Mom while tears rolled down my cheeks. Mom needed lots of love and comfort just like a child. I realized now that there was a role reversal. I was the parent and she was the child. I missed having a mother who took care of me, and that day I cried. My emotions were a combination of feeling so heartbroken for the anguish that my mother was experiencing, and also, I was saddened for my loss.

Mom was beginning to have more of these memory lapses. Many days she felt she was back in the Depression by the way she would ration her food. One of her favorite foods was Tastykakes lemon pie. I would bring her one every day. First she would break the pie in half and then break the half and only eat a quarter of the pie. She ended up eating the whole pie but felt she was only eating a quarter of it. One day I brought her a Hershey bar. She broke a little piece off and ate it. Then she said, "I'm going to save some for my brother, Gus."

"Oh Mom, you could eat the whole thing," I said. "If we see Uncle Gus, I have extra candy I could give him."

Mom absolutely adored her brother. He was a little younger than Mom. Growing up in a big family with seven siblings, she felt very protective of him. My Uncle Gus told stories of how much he loved chocolate candy when he was a kid. He would say once in a while, a relative would give each of the kids in the family a chocolate bar. It was a real treat. They all would just devour it right away. All except his sister, Francie. She stretched her candy bar out all week. Actually she only ate half because she waited to be alone with him and broke a piece off for the two of them to share.

Picturing this warmed my heart. Even as a child, my mother wanted to share with her brother. He was always so special to her. The two of them had such a strong bond since childhood.

22
Criticism Does No Good

As Alzheimer's disease progressed, Mom was losing her language skills. She often groped for the right word to use. She would refer to her husband as her father. She only saw Chuckie once a week but knew he was her son and tried to dote on him. She saw me every day, but I guess I annoyed her at times insisting that she keep up with her hygiene. Also, I was constantly criticizing Mom's speech. She felt I was so bossy.

Once as I was coming in, I heard her say to Dad, "Here comes that Pain in the Ass." Well, that felt like a real kick in the rear. Here I am doing everything possible for my parents, and my loving mother refers to me as that Pain in the Ass. Now how do you like that?

"Well, I guess she has a point," I said to myself. "Nobody likes being corrected, criticized, and told what to do," I said with a sigh. Then I remembered a phrase that I used quite a bit when I was parenting my two teenage daughters.

"Choose your battles wisely." Life is filled with opportunities to choose between making a big deal out of something or simply letting it go. I learned from being a parent that it is easy to get in the habit of fighting over the smallest things. When this occurs, there is so much frustration with everyone involved. A more peaceful way to live is to consciously decide which battles are worth fighting. Choosing my battles wisely could be applied to other aspects of my life. Now instead of parenting my daughters, I must parent my mother.

I tried making a conscious effort to stop criticizing Mom's mistakes in her speech. Did it really matter if she referred to her husband as her father? Or her wristwatch as the clock? I knew what she meant, and it served no purpose to point out her mistakes. It only made her defensive and lash out in anger. Other times it made her withdraw.

Sometimes Mom just could not think of the right word and would substitute a description for a specific object. Mom said things like, "Where's my . . . you know . . . my . . . the thing I put my money in."

"Do you want your pocketbook?" I would ask.

"Yeah, that's it," Mom would say.

I realized how frustrating it was for Mom to be unable to communicate properly. So I reevaluated my priorities. When the urge to criticize arose, I tried to catch myself. When Mom was having difficulty finding the correct word or expressing an idea, I supplied it for her. There was no point in having her struggle with lost vocabulary. I turned my criticism into understanding and tolerance. Now a touching moment came into my mind. Mom was struggling with the buttons on her coat.

"Let me help you with these buttons, Mom."

She looked at me and said, "You're always so good to me; it's like we're sisters." I just smiled. There was no use explaining to Mom that we were mother and daughter.

23
Life Keeps Changing

Life was fairly uneventful for the next couple months. I felt things were easier to handle. Dad was there to see that Mom did not wander away. She could still do things with simple instructions and was even able to help Dad. He had a hard time walking and getting out of a chair, but she could get what he needed. So the situation was workable.

Then came a big change. My father suffered from congestive heart failure and was hospitalized. There were a lot of complications with Dad's health. He ended up staying in the hospital and rehab for three months. Mom could not be in the apartment by herself. She had to stay with me again.

With every change of environment or lifestyle, Mom became more bewildered. She had to become familiar with my house again. She was much more confused than the last time she stayed with me. She did not want me out of her sight, and it even became a problem when the phone rang. Mom wanted my undivided attention and kept interrupting my phone conversations.

This was so ironic because I remember having this same problem with Denise when she was a toddler. Not knowing how to handle the situation, I discussed it with Mom. Mom's suggestion was to tell Denise that it is very important that you have this phone conversation but after you hang up, you will read her a story. I tried using the same principle on Mom. It worked as long as my conversations were not too long.

Also, Mom liked to follow me around the house and would become fretful if she did not know where I was, even for a short period of time.

"Where ya goin?" Mom would say with a bit of alarm in her voice.

"I have to go to the bathroom," I said.

"Why do you always have to go so much?" she asked.

"I don't know. I guess I'm one of those unusual people who have to go every five minutes," I said. Actually, I don't think I was exaggerating too much. Wherever I go, I must first find the bathroom. That may be my claim to fame.

Mom followed me to the bathroom. "I'll be right out," I said as I closed the door.

Mom waited by the door for about a minute before she said, "Ya done yet?"

"In a minute," I said.

This reminded me of when Denise and Krissy were toddlers. While they waited for me to come out of the bathroom, they would bang on the door. Maybe that's the reason I got into the habit of going so often. I was never able to complete whatever I was doing in there.

This behavior was getting me annoyed, but I tried to understand how Mom felt. Her world must seem so strange with constant memory lapses and a confused sense of time. She needed the security of being with a person whom she trusted to help her. So when I would close the door to the bathroom, I continued to talk to her in a reassuring way so she would not have that separation anxiety.

24
Praise Feels Good

Even though my mother's intellectual and physical capacity declined, she still maintained some skill and knowledge. Mom lost her ability to organize and plan her day's routine but with prompting, she could complete certain chores. If I wanted to take a quick shower, I would first give Mom a dust cloth and ask her if she would go around the room and dust the furniture. Not only was this a meaningful activity for Mom, but also it was helpful to me. While Mom was concentrating on this useful chore, I could shower without her panicking and banging on the door.

When Mom did a good job, I always praised her. Like everyone else, people afflicted with Alzheimer's still want to feel useful. As long as she could respond to activity at some level, I learned to devise ways to occupy her.

Like many memory-impaired people, Mom lost the ability to entertain herself. Self-amusement requires a memory for an extended period of time; unfortunately, Mom no longer had that capacity. However, she did not lose all ability to be amused. Mom was not capable of telling me what she liked but could respond when prompted.

As I was growing up, I remember Mom taking great pride in her flower garden. Every year she planted marigolds around a birdbath in the front lawn. On the side of the house, she grew beautiful tulips and in the backyard were her rose bushes. She loved to plant her flowers and watch them flourish. Watering the flowers would be an activity that Mom would enjoy.

"Mom, do you remember all the flowers you used to plant in our yard when we lived in our house on New Hope Street?" I asked.

"Yeah, I like to plant the flowers," she said.

"Everyone said your yard looked so beautiful. You really took very good care of the garden," I said. Mom's face lit up. I believe she remembered her lovely yard and longed for it.

"Would you like to help me take care of my flowers outside?" I asked.

"Okay," Mom said with enthusiasm.

We went outside, and I showed Mom the flowers and plants that needed watering. I no longer used my old stainless steel teakettle so I thought that would be easy for Mom to use while watering the plants. It had a handle and a spout and was not too heavy. I filled the kettle up with water and demonstrated how to water each plant. Then I gave the pail of water to Mom.

"Here Mom, now you try it."

She took the pail from me and proceeded to water each plant very carefully. I noticed that she made sure that the root of the plant got enough water. When the kettle was empty, I would refill it.

Mom and I got into a routine. Every evening when the sun went down, we enjoyed watering the flowers. When we would notice new buds blooming, we were delighted. Together we would admire our creation.

"Well Mom, you have that special touch with flowers. You're making the yard look like a beautiful picture," I said.

Mom beamed at the praise. Watering the flowers was a source of pleasure and comfort to her. This activity not only made her feel useful, but by the way she lovingly handled the plants, she retained some of her previous skill and knowledge about gardening. For me, this activity created a precious memory with my mother.

25
Adult Day Care Center

With both my parents in need of care, I needed some relief. One of the resources available for people suffering from dementia is Adult Day Care Centers. Day care is a viable alternative to institutionalizing loved ones. The day care center in our area had a staff of a director, nurse, social coordinator, and aids. I enrolled Mom for three days a week from 9:00 am to 3:00 pm.

She participated in the activities, games, and arts and crafts. She also participated in a program of reality orientation, which she was encouraged to know the day, date, month, year, and so forth. This was a good mental exercise, and I would try to reinforce the day care's efforts by continuing to use reality orientation in the evening when Mom was home with me.

Other programs included music therapy, which was used to evoke memories and emotions. Supervised exercises help to release energy and control the person's restlessness. Also, lunch was provided, and Mom had the opportunity to socialize with others in a safe environment.

Day care provided a well-needed respite for me. I had the opportunity to take care of Mom in my home without the burden of twenty-four hour care. Also, the day care is flexible to suit my needs and the needs of other caregivers in terms of hours and days per week. When full-time home care becomes too burdensome, day care can be a step before putting your loved one in a nursing home. Day care provides relief and is a bridge between the two types of care. They did have a van that would pick up Mom and take her back to my house at the end of the day, but I preferred driving. I had to ease into anything new. Mom had a little anxiety about going every day and being left there because she was afraid she would not get home. I always assured her that I would come back for her.

26
Repetitious Behavior

My mother would ask the same question over and over again. Or she would perform the same action over and over again. Mom's repetitious behavior could be extremely frustrating at times.

Every night before Mom went to bed, she laid out her clothes for the next day. Sometimes she would like to try on her outfit to make sure she was pleased with it. She tried on her slacks and top. Then she decided to try on another outfit. After the second outfit, she forgot she tried on the first one and put it on again. This led to a vicious cycle for hours.

"Mom, your clothes are fine," I said. "It's time to get into bed."

"Where's my socks?" she asked.

"Right here," I said.

"I don't see my shoes," she stated.

"Your shoes are right here by the bed," I assured her.

"Mom please get into bed," I pleaded. "I'm tired and need to sleep. I'm going to turn out the lights now."

"Wait a minute. I just want to try on my blouse before I get into bed," she said.

This is nowhere near the end, I thought. I was so tired and losing patience. I did not like to go to bed until Mom was in bed, but this night I had to make an exception.

"Mom, I'm going to bed now, and you go to bed whenever you're ready. I'll close the door in your room and you can keep on the light," I said.

Mom was trying clothes on for hours. It was so frustrating. I was also concerned about the rest of the family. Dom and Denise cannot be disturbed by this wandering and repetitious behavior at night. They both have to get up the next morning for work and school. It was 2:00 a.m. Finally, I got up. I guess Mom was tired or completely forgot what she was doing. I encouraged her to get into bed. I know one thing. I was not going to allow Mom to take a nap in the afternoon. She will just have to be tired during the day so that she will fall asleep at night.

As Alzheimer's disease progresses, the person will ask the same question over and over again. They could develop an obsession to the smallest detail. This repetition could be exhausting for the caregiver. The best way to approach the problem is with kindness and compassion. Mom needed reassurance to her repeated questions. By the repetitious behavior and questions she always asked gave me an indication about her concerns. The way Mom worried about her clothes was a clue that she still wanted to look nice. Mom never bought a lot for herself, but she valued what she had and took very good care of it. That habit was still with her.

Mom constantly asked the same questions. She was trying to figure out what changed in her life.

I remember taking Mom and Dad to my Aunt Fran and Uncle Bob's 50th anniversary party. Mom never wanted me out of her sight. I happened to go to the rest room. When I came back, Dom told me that Mom asked him countless times where I was. He assured her over and over again that I was coming back. Mom was afraid of being stranded without me.

27
Sense of Humor Needed

Some days I felt very good about the way I handled things, yet other times I regret being so abrupt. One morning it was very hard getting Mom ready and out the door to go to day care. We argued about what she was wearing. Mom decided then that she wanted to change her outfit, but we were running late.

"WE HAVE TO GO NOW!" I shouted as I was pulling on Mom's arm to get out the door. Finally, we got into the car and on our way, but we were both very angry. I left her at the day care and went about my daily routine. Three o'clock came quickly, and it was time for me to pick up Mom. When I got there, she was waiting for me.

On the ride home, Mom said, "I'm so glad you came for me instead of that other lady that took me this morning. That lady is so mean. What's wrong with her?"

I smiled and just agreed with Mom.

"Oh that other lady is mean. Everybody says that about her. She's a real bitch."

Then Mom and I just giggled about that bitchy lady. Laughing at the situation and myself helped ease the tension and made this life's journey less difficult.

A sense of humor gives you resilience. It keeps you from

getting too serious when things do not go your way. Sometimes a sense of humor is the only way to get through the day.

The comedian Bill Cosby once said, "If you can find humor in something, you can survive it."

28
Negative Thoughts

Another emotion that I had to learn to deal with was fear. Negative thoughts were constantly coming into my mind. My imagination would run away with me, and I would drum up every possible situation. This leads to generalized worry.

How bad is this illness going to get? Will Mom lose all quality to life? Will she suffer? Am I going to get Alzheimer's?

In the past, my personality has been to harbor fears so intensely that it has manifested itself with anxiety. The things I fear do not even need to happen; it already has—or it might as well have—because I am forcing myself to live through it.

Now I cannot blame my emotions of worry and anxiety entirely on Mom's illness. I have been a worrier for as long as I could remember. In fact, I have lived with worry for so long that it actually is hard to recognize as anything out of the ordinary. Worry serves no purpose in helping the situation. I am aware that in my past, worry and anxiety have robbed me of daily energy and the ability to live with confidence. On the flip side, I believe I inherited this trait from "Good Ol Mom."

I must turn these negative emotions around and not allow my future concerns to dominate the present moments. These emotions of fear, worry, and anxiety start with a conscious decision. It has always been very easy for me to become tangled up in a web of negativity without ever realizing that this is a choice. Thoughts could have great power over a person. My thoughts are followed by feelings such as anger, jealousy, and fear, which then lead to unhappiness. It is impossible to have this sadness without first having the thought that produces these emotions. Unhappiness simply cannot exist alone. It must be accompanied by negative thoughts.

However after a lifetime of this debilitating habit, I needed to take control of my thinking. It became essential that I practice positive thinking. After making this decision, I cannot say that I eliminated all negative thoughts, but I learned to choose what to do with them. When I feel upset, I immediately take notice of my thinking and remind myself that it is my thoughts that are negative, not my life.

When I thought of my mother's illness progressing in the future to the point of her becoming incontinent, my first reaction was to feel upset. However, dwelling on this negative thought serves absolutely no purpose. It helped to remind myself that if the situation gets overwhelming for me, I have the option of putting Mom in a skilled nursing home. Then I would dismiss the negative thought and replace it with a positive one.

Also, I am learning to stay in the present moment. It is so overwhelming to always be anticipating the future. How tiring it is to think about all that needs to be done along with the potential problems and responsibilities. Also, it is just as exhausting to dwell on the mistakes and imperfect results of the past. When our minds linger too long on the past and future, it can spoil the moment we are in now. During my caregiving experience, I am learning to stay in the immediate moment. This takes effort. Many times I needed to remind myself to come back to the present. Then the future will fall into place.

29
Taking Care of Me

During this part of my life's journey, I learned to recognize that I am human and naturally have weak points. I am most vulnerable to feeling depressed when I am lonely or tired. If I keep pushing past my limits, I create more stress. Some warning signs for me are my neck and shoulders ache. This tells me I am tense and overworked. Then it is hard to concentrate on what needs to be done. My mind starts racing, and I make a lot of little mistakes like misplacing my keys and eyeglasses. So much time is wasted looking for them. I may forget an ingredient while preparing dinner. On a more serious note, while rushing around so much, I have gotten a few fender benders while driving. Then sadness comes over me, and the negative events in my life are exaggerated in my own mind. When this happens, it is easy to forget that anything good has ever occurred, and I start to think I am a complete failure. That is when I need to take responsibility for taking care of myself.

During these vulnerable times, several strategies are helpful. I keep a gratitude journal by writing down all the positive qualities and events in my life. This forces me to realize my good fortune and get a clearer perspective on my situation. At the top of my journal is a supportive husband

and independent daughters. Also on my list are good health and prosperity.

Although it is heartbreaking to watch Mom's mental decline, I feel very thankful that we shared an extremely close mother-daughter bond. I learned that it is not a relationship that everyone has. After jotting down all these positives, I was amazed to see a very long list. During my caregiving experience, referring to this gratitude journal often was helpful. I was able to change my focus. Focusing my attention on what I have instead of what I want gave me a brighter outlook on life.

Another tactic in taking care of me is learning relaxation techniques. Your mind and body end up being one. If you have mental tension, it eventually results in a muscular tension. Learning to relax is a powerful tool to diffuse the tension that your body builds up in response to the emotional turmoil that worry, anger, and frustration can cause.

Here are some of the relaxation exercises I do. It only takes ten minutes a day but does a world of good. I try to get as comfortable as I can and take a deep breath. I hold it for ten seconds and then exhale slowly. This is repeated three times. Immediately, a calmer feeling comes over me. Then I tense the muscles in my body at one time and hold this rigid form. After about five seconds, I relax the muscles. The tension leaves me and my body feels limp and relaxed.

During this relaxed state, I picture the waves breaking in the ocean. While creating this mental picture, other senses are used to hear the roar of the ocean and to smell the fragrance of salt water. Cares and concerns seem to float away in this state of tranquility.

Also when feeling sad, I learned to avoid individuals who feel the need to criticize my weaknesses. This is the time I especially need to be with people who are understanding. Joining a support group for the family of a person suffering from dementia is helpful. Support groups are composed of people who have lived through the experience of having a family member with Alzheimer's or are presently faced with this situation. The group shares the collective wisdom of managing this illness.

Every caregiver should attend a support group for many reasons. In the early stages of the disease, the caregiver will gain knowledge. As the illness progresses, the caregiver and the impaired relative can become more isolated. The support group becomes the only place where the caregiver receives a sense of positive reinforcement.

Also, he or she could express discomforting feelings in an accepting and confidential environment. For example, group members understand the internal conflicts of caregivers. You may express feelings of abandoning your loved one. At the same time, look for renewed strength to maintain quality to the memory impaired person's life. There is an experiential understanding of the unfairness of Alzheimer's disease and comfort in shared tragedy.

For a short respite, I walked around the block in my neighborhood. This was always refreshing. When I started walking, I joined other people and developed some wonderful friendships. My new friend Elaine had a similar situation with aging parents. As we walked, we shared stories and helpful information. We vented our frustrations and were sympathetic listeners to each other without feeling judged.

In addition to having friends who have similar problems, it is equally important to be around people who are upbeat, positive, and energetic. They could act as role models and their attitude could be enticing. I depend on my friend Marene for this. It is so important for the caregiver to maintain friendships.

The caregiver must always be aware if he or she is becoming too isolated. This is the time to be assertive and contact friends. It does take energy especially if you are exhausted. You may even experience a feeling of guilt for enjoying yourself with friends; but it is so necessary to preserve your own mental and physical health.

Also, caregivers need to keep up with their medical and dental checkups. More than 1 in 10 caregivers become physically ill or injured as a result of caregiving; anywhere from 43% to 46% suffer from depression.[33] A study published in the *Proceedings of the National Academy of Sciences* concluded that the stress of caring for your loved one at home can prematurely age the immune system. This puts caregivers at risk of developing additional age related illnesses.[34]

Since each person is different, he or she will have different levels of tolerance and different ways of responding to a problem. To avoid unhealthy habits, the caregiver should take a self-inventory once a week by asking him or herself some questions.

Am I unusually sad? Do I cry easily? Am I anxious? Am I staying awake at night worrying about the situation? Am I losing weight? Am I medicating myself by overeating, smoking, or alcohol abuse? Do I need tranquilizers to get through the day? Do I feel isolated? Do I have feelings of resentment? Do I lash out in anger? Do I take my anger out on the impaired person?

Since we are all human, it is normal to feel overwhelmed at times. However, if you are saying yes to most of these questions, you need to seek help. Asking yourself these questions will help you stay aware of your well-being which will enable you to stay in control of your life.

30
Childish Ways

There were times my mother was reverting back to childish ways. One evening after we went to the hospital to visit Dad, we went for a bite to eat. We had pizza. I ordered Mom her coffee, and I had a diet coke.

"What are you drinking?" Mom asked.

"Soda," I said.

"Well, how come I don't have one?" she snapped.

"You always get coffee," I said.

We continued eating but Mom did not look happy.

"Is everything good?" I asked.

"NO!" she said. "I want what you have."

"Mom, you never drink soda. That's why I didn't get you one," I said.

"You got one for yourself. You just didn't want to get me one," she stated indignantly.

"Here. Here's my soda. Are you happy now?" I snapped.

She took my soda and had a smug look on her face. She wasn't going to let anyone fool her. I just sighed with exasperation.

Another incident I remember was when Mom and I got into the car with a bag of groceries. She saw the Tastykake lemon pie that she loved so much on top of the bag.

"I want a piece of that," she said.

"When we get home, you can eat it," I said.

"Let's eat it now. That way we won't have to share it with all the others," she said.

I had to smile. Mom thought she was back in the Depression living in a big family where she never got enough.

I just said, "Mom, you can eat that whole pie when we get home. I am on a diet so I don't want any, and the only one home is Dad. He just wants his cigarettes."

That seemed to pacify her. It was only a short ride home but like a child, Mom wanted instant gratification.

She kept asking, "We home yet? Did you get lost? How long is it gonna be?" Finally we are home, but Mom did not take her eyes off that lemon pie.

31
Suspicious Behavior

Some days I would get up early to get a head start on my list of things to do. I got so much more accomplished while Mom was still in bed. I decided to throw in a load of laundry while grading the essays from the ninth grade class. I quietly tiptoed into Mom's room to pick up her clothes from the hamper.

After the last essay was graded and the clothes were in the dryer, I got Mom up and started her routine. As I was helping Mom get dressed, she felt the need to confide in me.

"Ya know that lady who lives across the hall," she said as she was pointing to my bedroom. Mom was confused and thought this was an apartment building.

"Yeah, what about her?" I asked.

"She has some nerve," Mom said.

"Why? What did she do?" I asked.

"Well, she just walks right in my house while I'm in bed and steals my clothes," she said with contempt. "**Can you believe that woman?**"

I guess Mom saw me coming into her room this morning rummaging through her clothes. It was useless to reason with Mom so I tried to pacify her.

"Mom, I think that woman just borrowed some clothes. She'll give them back," I said.

"But that's not right," she stated with indignation. "She just walks right in and takes my panties without even asking. Doesn't she have any of her own?"

I had to smile at how ridiculous this conversation was.

Then Mom blurted out with a sense of justice, "How bout if I just walked into her house and took her panties? Would she like it?"

"Oh, that woman would be furious if someone did that to her," I said.

"Well, she has some damn nerve," Mom stated.

"Stealing someone's panties is about as low as you get," I said acknowledging Mom's indignation. Then I tried to change the subject.

Victims of Alzheimer's have a tendency to be suspicious of others. They also suffer from delusions and hallucinations. An Alzheimer sufferer might worry about someone stealing from him or her. The person often hides possessions. When unable to find these belongings, the forgetful individual may accuse close relatives and friends of stealing. It is useless to try to argue with a memory-impaired person out of his or her false beliefs. Assure your loved one that you are there for him or her and then offer a distraction from the situation.

Many times the caregiver becomes the target of blame for these imagined evils. It is natural for the caregiver to react to the suspicions of the confused relative by feeling hurt. Anger wells up and the caregiver may feel abused by these false accusations.

If this situation occurs, remember that the accusations stem from fear. A person suffering from Alzheimer's does not have the ability to test reality. For an individual who cannot remember what happened an hour ago or even who he or she is, there is no place to feel safe. This overwhelming feeling of loss causes the confused person to feel vulnerable. An Alzheimer's patient is struggling to make sense of nonsense in a world that is foreign and frightening. Your loved one needs your reassurance when these episodes occur.

32
Simplify Meal Time

On holidays, I learned it is better to simplify dinners and festivities as much as possible. When our family sat down for Easter dinner, Mom seemed very confused at the big variety on the table. She did not know what to do. I came to her rescue and asked if she would like me to fix her plate. She agreed and looked relieved.

As I learned to adjust to Mom's needs, I limited the variety on the plate. Also, I would cut the food into small pieces so she could pick it up easily. Then only one utensil was necessary at Mom's place setting. It was best not to put salt and pepper shakers on the table. Mom would forget she salted her food and would do it over and over again. I started fixing Mom's coffee for her; otherwise, she poured in the sugar. That was another odd thing. Before Mom's illness, she never took sugar in her coffee. Now her sweet tooth seemed to be insatiable.

I was more comfortable with Mom using a plastic cup and plate. It was better not to fill the glass to its capacity. There were a lot fewer accidents. It was easier to serve most meals in the kitchen where I could easily clean up the floor if something dropped. Simplifying mealtime is essential. The hands and the brain of a person suffering from Alzheimer's no longer work together. The impaired individual may understand what he or she wants to do, but the message does not connect from the brain to the hands.

Also, it is important to watch your loved one for dehydration. Dehydration in an Alzheimer patient is very common. They simply do not know when they are thirsty. Many times they will rely on caffeinated drinks such as coffee, tea, or soda. Mom always enjoyed her coffee, but I tried to limit her intake to the early part of the day. Caffeine acts as a diuretic and could contribute to dehydration.

The best thirst quencher is water. I tried to always have a plastic cup of water in front of Mom. Seeing the cup would remind her to take a sip.

33
Enlightenment

During this journey through life, I not only learned about Alzheimer's disease and how to handle Mom, but I discovered a great deal about myself. Each crisis or situation caused me to reevaluate my outlook on life. For as long as I could remember, I was a perfectionist.

For example, Dom and I love having our friends over, and we entertain often. I take pride in my gourmet hors d'oeuvres and fabulous desserts. When I receive company, my house must be spotless and seasonally decorated with scented candles burning in various rooms. I usually invite small groups because only six people could sit comfortably around our dining room table. I even go as far as mixing friends whom I feel have something in common so that everyone will get along and feel some connection.

Here is an example of my planning strategy for a perfect evening.

During this Christmas season, I think I will invite Theresa and Dave Leach with Sandy and Lou Corsi. They are both planning weddings for their daughters so they should be compatible. What about Marene and Dave? They might enjoy talking to Janet and John. Oh No! Maybe Marene and Dave would be more compatible with Marcy and Ernie. Now, I think Anita and Ron would enjoy

*Ruth and Bob Travaglini. Both Ruth and Anita are very involved
with raising teenagers. They could share stories while Bob and Ron
will probably talk about their work.*

Then I choose some dates to receive my company and get
on the phone to make arrangements. Sometimes that requires
juggling people and dates to accommodate everyone. When I
have these small groups, the evening always goes well, and I
am proud of myself for my hosting ability. But, this is no easy
task. After all this cleaning, decorating, food preparation, and
strategically grouping my guests, I am exhausted.

This Christmas season with my time-consuming
responsibility of taking care of my parents, the thought of
entertaining was depleting my energy. But I still felt I needed a
diversion from my normal routine. I wanted to be with my
friends and have some fun. This was when I realized that I was
trapped by perfectionism. The pressure that I put on myself
needed adjusting. So I thought about this trait of perfectionism
and decided it was causing me misery instead of joy.

This idea of perfectionism consumes so much of my life. I
cannot blame this one on my mother because when I was
growing up, our house was never perfect. However, I truly
believed we were the only family who did not fit that image.
Since television was a big part of entertainment during my
impressionable years, I am going to give 'June Cleaver' from
"Leave It To Beaver" the credit for my neurotic insistence of
perfectionism. There were many other television characters
such as 'Donna Stone' from "The Donna Reed Show" and
'Laura Petri' from "The Dick Van Dyke Show" reinforcing my
quest for this picture-perfect life.

In my early years, I believe 'June Cleaver' was the most
influential. Her house was the epitome of perfection, and she
did this with so little effort. I can still picture 'Mrs. Cleaver' in
her high heels and pearls while icing her freshly baked cake.
There were no dirty dishes around or dough splattered on the
floor or table—not even a utensil out of place.

As I got older, I graduated to the soap operas. Soap opera characters had such dysfunctional lives, but their homes were beautifully decorated. Even the actors' outfits coordinated well with the furniture. I started thinking about this fantasy image presented by the media and how it consumed my life in so many ways. I actually started to feel foolish.

Gee, I thought, *I am not even emulating a real person. I am putting so much effort into creating an image.*

Then I made a decision. Perfection is unattainable. I will just do my best. I gave myself permission to cut corners. Instead of making refreshments, I bought them. Then there was less cleaning to do in the kitchen. I invited some friends without thinking of who would be compatible. Many of them have different interests, but we all have one thing in common. We all know about aging parents. When I adjusted my attitude, the pressure was off me, and I began to relax.

The evening turned out great even with my store bought refreshments. The table was a little crowded because eight people sat around this time. Janet and John Lisa were a wealth of knowledge with their traveling. Marene and Dave came. Being a high school teacher, Dave had amusing stories to share with us. Then, the Leach's showed up, and the gathering really got lively. Theresa is one of those people who is always in a crisis. However, when she talks about her catastrophes, it comes out comical. The evening was livelier than ever with everyone sharing his or her different interests and stories.

Lessons are learned when you least expect them. This Christmas season I discovered how much of my life is spent living up to a standard that is impossible to achieve. I now consciously strive to do my best but accept that perfection is unattainable. And why would anyone even want it? Perfection does not leave much room for acceptance and joy. Our imperfections make us interesting and exciting. On a final note, I think anyone who is as perfect as 'June Cleaver' is a bore.

34
Comparisons

As I continued to see my caregiving as an opportunity to grow, I thought about some of my other tendencies. Even though I hate to admit it, I was constantly comparing myself to others. "She has more education."

"She has a high-powered job."

"Her life is so exciting." The list goes on and on. Of course, when a woman covets the looks of the models and actresses, she is sure to come up feeling inferior.

Farrah Fawcett in "Charlie's Angels" has always been my standard for beauty. Now I know that even Farrah has aged, but I still continue to picture her with the physical characteristics she had in her twenties—great figure, flawless complexion, and of course, her trademark, the hair. Envying these attributes did not leave me much room to appreciate who I was. I was my own worst enemy. I knew I had to give up on these comparisons if I was going to achieve peace of mind and happiness.

However, being a caregiver gave me a complete new outlook on life. By tackling each problem that arose each day, I was gaining self-confidence and a strength that I did not know I had. So I decided that I did not have to compare myself to others. I also acknowledged what I probably already knew.

Much of what is presented by the media is the airbrushed, computerized version of what appears to be the real person.

I needed to appreciate myself for who I was. So I started looking within and discovered I was proud of the job I was doing in caring for my parents. It was a tremendous learning experience and an opportunity to grow. I was gaining peace of mind and self-confidence.

In the end, a woman's beauty exudes when she feels good inside. Always looking outward promotes envy, frustration, and a lack of satisfaction. So right then I decided to turn off the "Fawcett." This million-dollar industry was no longer going to rule my life. I recognized that I was being the best I could, and all I needed to do is measure up to my own internal yardstick. I still admire the wonderful qualities of others, but I feel content with me.

35
Faced with Decisions

My father had been in two hospitals and rehab for about three months after suffering from congenital heart failure. For the last three weeks, he was in a rehab for physical therapy. At this point, the insurance would no longer cover his stay. Dad looked very weak and had aged quite a bit during this time, but therapy would no longer be available for him. Mom and I visited him every day in the hospital and the rehab. He lost a lot of weight. He was depressed and did not have much of an appetite. We would bring him homemade dinners and goodies to entice him into eating. While going back and forth to the rehab, I got to know the workers and administration. I would go to meetings discussing Dad's progress and sometimes his uncooperative behavior. He did not want to be there. Even though he looked very frail and weak, he said, "I have nothing in common with all these old people."

Three days before Dad's release, the administration called me in for a meeting with the business administrator, nursing director, and social services representative. They knew the situation with Mom. I sat there in the office listening to their very strong arguments that my mother and father should not go back to the apartment.

The nursing director June said, "Mrs. DiPaolo, your dad is

not going to be able to take care of himself, let alone handle your mother. And your mother certainly can't take care of your dad."

"I know that," I acknowledged. "It has been that way for a couple of years now."

The business director Diane chimed in and said, "We know you are doing the best you can, but wouldn't it be more practical if your mother and father lived in our nursing facility." She continued to explain, "We could arrange that the two of them could share a room together. It would take a lot of pressure off of you."

Then June said, "Your parents would still be together. They would get their meals and medication. And someone would always be here in case they needed help."

"Well, I have thought about placing my parents in a nursing home, but I am not sure we are ready just yet," I said tentatively.

Diane argued, "It's really not fair for you to spend so much time with your parents when you have your own family and life. And yet, your parents deserve to be safe."

Their argument was making sense to me. It was a lot to take in, and I knew I had to make a decision soon. Dad was going to be released from the rehab in three days.

Then Marlene the social director commented, "We see that your mother is in good physical shape and likes to follow you around. You could come and take your mother for a walk every day. Or you could take your parents for a ride or back to your house for dinner whenever you want. It's not like they would have to stay here 24-hours a day. You could still do the same things with them only you would know that they are safe," she said.

Then I asked about the financial part of this nursing facility. To be a resident in this nursing home was $4,500 a month per person, plus you must pay for your medications and some other incidentals. So I did a quick calculation and came up with approximately $10,000 a month. Then I asked if there would be a discount since both my parents would be residents sharing a room.

Diane said, "Unfortunately, we do not have a discount policy." She proceeded to tell me about the forms that I would have to fill out disclosing all of their assets. When their savings are reduced to $2000, they will then be eligible for Medicaid.

What a shame it was that my mother and father were so frugal all of their lives. I would have felt so much better if they had used some of this money to go on a nice vacation.

All this information and the decisions I faced were making me feel overwhelmed. I took a deep breath and said, "I'm going to have to give this some serious thought."

They all agreed that it was a good idea for me to go home and think about our discussion.

I thought about this for the rest of the day, and when Dom came home I discussed it with him. If my mother and father would go back to live in their apartment, Dad was going to require more help. I would have to be with them most of the day. Also, I would still have to make sure Chuckie is doing well. I now attend meetings in his behalf. I would still want to drive Chuckie over to visit Mom and Dad once a week. I was responsible for three people. After we thoroughly mulled it over, we still did not come up with a solution. Dom said, "Hon, whatever you decide, I will be supportive."

I also talked to my aunt about the situation.

"Aunt Anna, what do you think I should do?" I asked.

My aunt looked very concerned as she said, "So far, you have been able to handle this. But it is going to be a big change now that your father needs more help. I don't like the idea of them being in a nursing home, but I don't want to see you get so run down and end up getting sick."

I was still in a dilemma. No one was too much help in convincing me which way to go.

The next day when Mom and I went to visit Dad in the rehab, I told him about the meeting that I had with the administration.

"Dad, the staff feels that you and Mom would be better off living here. They were telling me that the two of you really should not be on your own at all. You can't walk very well and you're so weak. Do you think you and Mom would like to live here?" I asked.

"ARE YOU CRAZY? WHY WOULD I WANT TO LIVE HERE WITH ALL THESE OLD PEOPLE?" he stated adamantly. "I WANNA GET OUTTA HERE."

Isn't that just like my father? He could barely walk. He couldn't do much for himself. But he did not include himself as one of these old people.

"But Dad, what would happen if you would get up in the middle of the night and fall?" I asked. "Nobody would be there who could help you."

"I don't get up in the middle of the night," he said. So as far as he was concerned, we did not have a problem. He hated being in the rehab and couldn't wait to go home.

I thought about the positives and negatives in this situation. For the rest of the day, I had an internal argument with myself.

Being the primary caregiver was becoming more than a full time job. What if there was a snowstorm, and I could not get to Mom and Dad one day? There would always be a staff available at the nursing home. I would have so much freedom. But I probably would be at the nursing home much of the time. The cost is astronomical. This is not how my parents expected to use their life savings. Mom and Dad would be safe living in the nursing home. But I know they would not flourish or feel comfortable. Dad never participated in any of the activities that were available in the rehab. He never even spent time with the other residents. He hated being there and longed to be back in his own place.

I went to sleep that night not being able to decide what was best for my parents. When I woke up the next morning, I still had the dilemma. All this intellect, assessment, and logic were confusing me more. Instead of relying on my head, I might be better off listening to my intuition—that inner voice guided by my heart.

I know my parents better than anyone. My intuition is telling me that my mother and father should stay together in their own apartment where they are comforted by familiarity. They have a better chance of thriving and living to their fullest capacity with me guiding them over each obstacle.

Maybe it is not always the head that sees clearly. Relying solely on your intellect or logic could result in making a decision based on fear. After thinking with my heart, the situation became clearer, and I am at peace with my decision. The heart is a balance for the mind and emotions. I took into account all that needed to be done and how to accomplish this. I would continue to be my parent's primary caregiver.

This may not be the answer for everyone. Each individual is different with every situation being unique. I am going to trust my intuition and follow my heart. In this journey of discovery, I learned that my inner voice has value. If I still have doubt after exhausting all logic and intellect, I need to listen to my heart.

36
Prioritizing Life

Dad was released from the rehab, and Mom went back to the apartment with him. For the next couple of weeks, I was there most of the day. By this time, I did not feel that I could give 100% to my part time job and also be the primary caregiver of my parents. I have never been one of those super achievers who could have it all and do it all. Even though some women say that they can, I am not sure it is possible without sacrificing something, especially your own health. I am the type of woman who feels you could have it all, just not at the same time. I love my job and it is great having extra money, but at this point, I feel overwhelmed with responsibility.

So I asked myself, "What is really important?" Despite the multitude of responsibilities, there is a choice of what is really important in my life. Asking myself this question helped me decide where I needed to put my greatest amount of energy. For me, the answer was simple. I had to give up my job. Even though this strategy seems overly simplistic, prioritizing what is really important kept me on track.

37
Scheduling the Routine

With both of my parents needing care, things had to change. In order for them to live in their home, they needed more help. To make matters worse, Dad could no longer drive. Although I was the primary caregiver, I could not do it all myself. I had to seek and accept whatever help I could get. Many times relatives and friends do not know how they could help so it is best to ask them specifically for what is needed.

Fortunately, Dad had great veteran's benefits. I had to go through a lot of bureaucracy, but I finally was able to get an aid to come in for ten hours a week. I set up a schedule and routine that was doable for my parents to live in their own surroundings. I went every morning to shower Mom and get her dressed. Dad got up on his own and was able to get dressed. Then, we went to Jems for brunch. They always went to the same diner because they liked familiarity. Mom and Dad also like to be served by the same waitresses Maureen, Rebecca, and Karen who knew the situation and always took care of them.

After brunch, we would do errands like banking, doctors' appointments, and shopping. Sometimes we would go to the market and buy groceries for dinner. Many times I bought already prepared food. Then about 3:00 p.m., I would take them back to the apartment. I started putting their dinner in plates and left it in the refrigerator. Then I wrote the instructions for the aid. That usually included showering my father and seeing that he put on clean clothes.

After Dad's hygiene was completed, the aid would heat up their dinner in the microwave and see that they ate. She was able to leave while they were eating but would put out finger food so they could snack all evening while they watched television. My parents were able to get ready and into bed themselves. Then they waited for me to come the next morning. Most of the time the dishes were still on the table so the first thing I would do was clear the table and wash the dishes. Next I retrieved their clothes from the hamper and put it in a laundry bag to take to my house. It was easier to combine their wash with mine. Then we started the routine all over again.

Since I had to be with my parents most of the day, I stopped taking Mom to day care. So now I took care of my mother and father with the help of the aid.

When I needed a break to go away for a few days, Aunt Anna watched over them. Also, I invested in a monitor that people wear around their necks. It is hooked up to the phone. If the individual wearing the monitor should fall or need help, all he or she has to do is press the button. The people working at the helpline are alerted and call back. If they do not get an answer, they will call relatives or the police to check on them. So that is how we managed.

Respite Care - I never used respite care but looked into it. Respite care is temporary residential programs. This allows the caregiver to place the patient in a special facility for a brief time. I was glad there was this program available in case I needed it.

38
Touch Therapy

Mom's language skills diminished to the point where it was difficult for her to verbally communicate. This was an additional burden because I had to respond to her needs without clear communications. My mother was getting more isolated and withdrawn. This was when I found that nonverbal communication could be quite powerful. I looked for physical signs—facial expressions and eye movements are ways in which I interpreted Mom's wants and needs.

Touch therapy is so important for anyone who is feeling isolated. I believe many elderly people would benefit from this type of human contact. I could tell that both my mother and father needed this. Holding Mom's arm while walking was comforting. Massaging Dad's neck and back while he was sitting in his chair would soothe him. Sometimes Mom would complain of aches and pains when she was going to bed.

She would say, "I feel sick."

My intuition told me that these pains were psychosomatic. She probably felt sick because she was afraid. Because of Mom's confusion with time, I believe she thought she had to go to school the next day. I rubbed Mom's neck and assured her that she was safe, and I was going to take care of her. I told her to just relax as I gently massaged her back. I would feel her muscles loosening and the anxiety leaving her body. Mom then felt comforted and would say, "I feel so good."

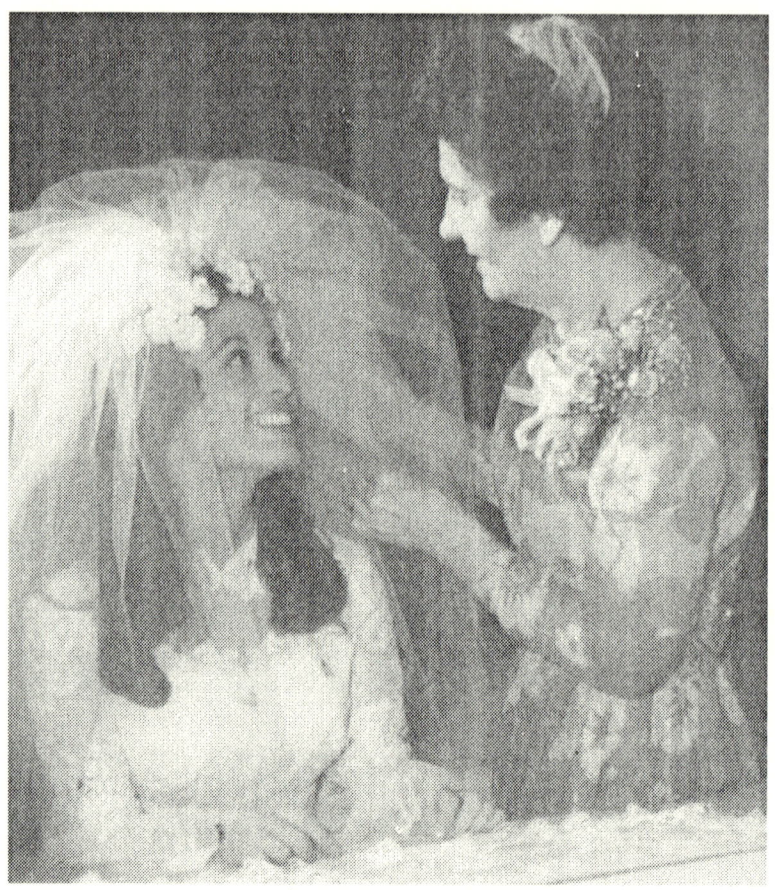

Mom and Daughter on wedding day

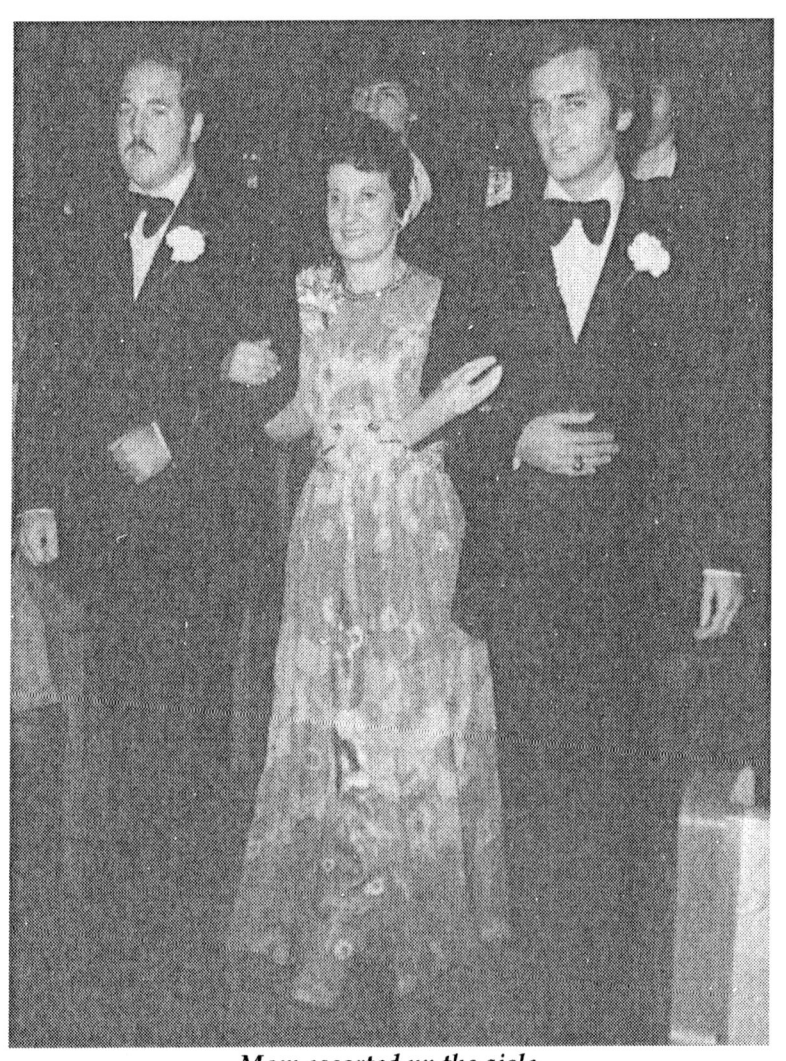

Mom escorted up the aisle

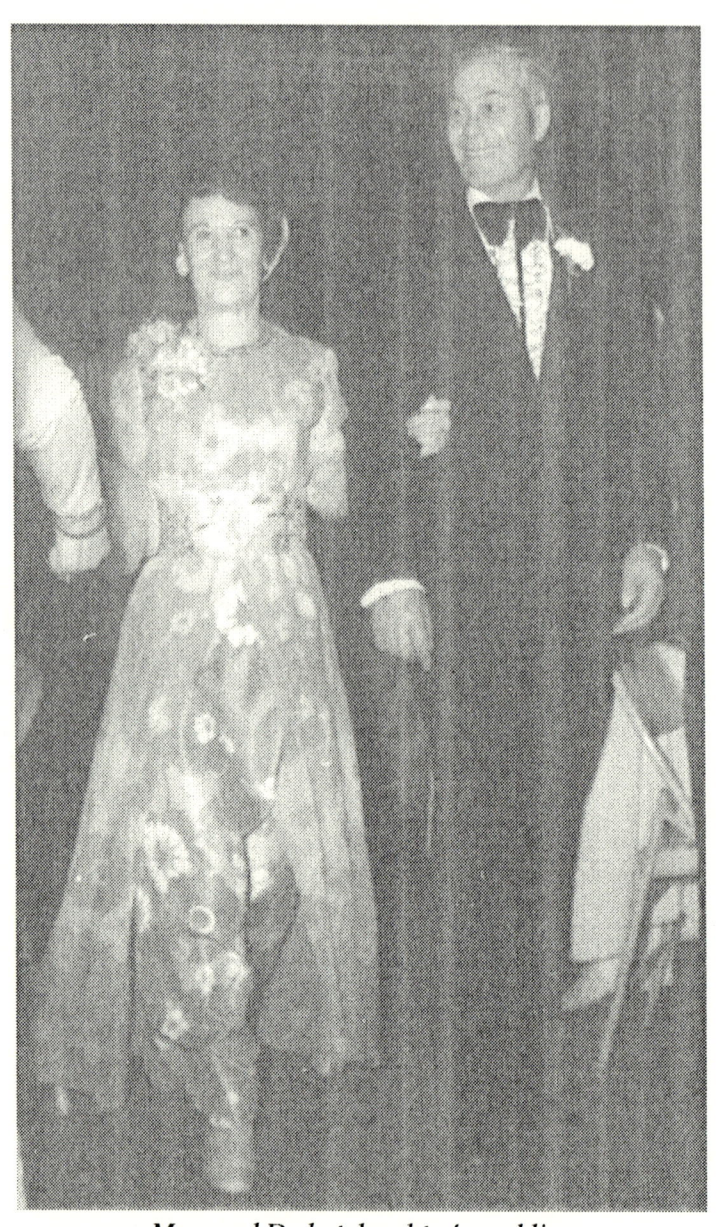

Mom and Dad at daughter's wedding

39
Activities

Mom now had such a short attention span that it was very hard to think of any activities to hold her interest. The television was always on, but I am not sure she focused on the program. I encouraged her to practice writing her name, but I noticed that she was having trouble. I would write it on a piece of paper first and then see if she could copy the letters. It was getting hard to determine her letter formation. Folding clothes was a chore that she could do, and at least she had the feeling of accomplishment.

One activity that Mom and I enjoyed doing together was looking at photo albums. Actually, I got just as much pleasure out of this. I had not looked at my wedding album in years. There were priceless memories in that album.

"Mom, look at you and Dad," I said. They both looked so healthy and vibrant.

"Do you remember your dress?" I asked.

"Is that me?" she asked.

"It certainly is," I said. "You were the mother of the bride. Here you are again fixing my veil."

"I like that dress," Mom said.

"Actually, it's been 28 years, and that dress is still hanging in your closet. It's very faded, but you never wanted to get rid of it. You always said you might wear it again when Denise or Kristen get married."

I remember getting a bit annoyed at Mom for even thinking that she would wear the dress at her granddaughter's wedding. Mom was always so frugal but that seemed ridiculous. "I don't think so," I said. "You could certainly afford a new dress as the Grandmother of the Bride."

Where did the time go, I thought? I remember shopping with Mom for my big day. I actually found my bridal gown rather quickly. But Mom was a little more of a problem. She looked at the mother of the bride gowns at the boutiques and thought everything looked too matronly. So we decided to look in the city. Mom and I took the train into Philadelphia on the hottest day in June. After looking in several stores, we found this shop on Chestnut Street that seemed to have dresses for special occasions.

"Let's go in here, Mom," I said.

"Okay, at least we'll be out of the heat for a while," Mom said.

We both started looking through the racks of dresses. We looked at each other and Mom whispered, "These prices are outrageous."

I had to agree. I knew Mom would never spend this kind of money on a dress. We were ready to leave the store when we spotted a rack of long dresses that were on sale.

The saleswoman said, "These gowns are reduced because they are discontinued. We will not be able to order any of them in different sizes."

Then we spotted the printed chiffon gown.

"Mom, this is your style," I pointed out.

She looked at it and said, "It is elegant." Then Mom looked at the price and said, "They may have drastically reduced this, but the price is still outrageous."

"Well, just try it on and see what it looks like," I said. I was starting to get impatient. "We haven't had much luck in finding anything."

"All right," she said, "I might as well see what it looks like."

When she tried it on, it was not exactly love at first sight. It was a little loose on her and much too long. She came out of the dressing room to look in a full-length mirror. The saleswoman said, "Try these heels on with the gown."

It looked better without it dragging on the floor, but it still was too big. The saleswoman said if we were interested in purchasing the dress, there was a woman who did alterations for the shop. We then put some pins on the seams to get the effect.

"I like it," I said. "It's perfect for you."

I could see the idea of buying the dress was starting to grow on Mom. "It will look great after the alterations," I said.

"Yeah, but it is ridiculous to pay this price," she said.

"Well Mom, it's not going to be easy finding you a gown. It's never easy finding anything for you," I said. "The way I see it, we've got two problems. You have a petite figure. So in your size, most of the shops have styles that cater to teenagers. You don't want to dress like a teeny bopper while you are escorted down the aisle."

Mom nodded in acknowledgment that it was hard to find appropriate apparel for her.

"The other problem," I continued, "you are cheap."

"I AM NOT CHEAP!" she retorted. "I have to be a bit practical about this. I'm only going to wear it one day," she said.

"Mom, you're the mother of the bride. It's going to be your only time," I pleaded.

"I don't know," she said. "Let me think about it. People are suppose to look at you that day, not me," she chuckled.

"Why don't you put some money down on the dress so the shop will hold it for you? We could still look around for a couple more days to see if we could find anything else," I said.

Mom agreed to do that only after the saleswoman assured her that she would be able to get her deposit back if she changed her mind.

We left the store relieved that we had a possibility. As we walked up the street looking for other shops, I reached in my pocketbook to get out some chewing gum.

"Want some gum, Mom?" I asked as I handed her a stick of Doublemint. Mom took the gum, broke a little piece off, and handed it back to me.

"You could have the whole piece," I said. I don't think I ever saw my mother chew a whole piece of gum. Whenever she wanted some, she would break a little bit off and save the rest. A pack of gum would last her so long that the last piece she chewed would be stale.

"I don't like putting a whole piece in my mouth," she said.

I just started to laugh at Mom's frugal ways. Looking at the wedding album with Mom today was causing me to think of the oddest things. I am so glad she decided to buy that gown. We really did not find anything else that suited her. After the alterations, the dress was perfect. Mom looked lovely.

I believe that gown was the most expensive outfit she ever bought for herself. I always kidded Mom about being cheap, but actually the only person she was cheap with was herself. Unfortunately, she never felt she was worth these luxuries. Growing up so poor and believing she was so unattractive gave her a very little sense of worth.

I remember when Mom was just diagnosed with Alzheimer's; I was trying to help her in the apartment. I was changing the sheets when I noticed a new set in the linen closet. The sheets and pillowcases were still in the original wrapping. I decided to use the new linens.

As I was opening the package, Mom started yelling, "Leave those alone. I'm saving them."

"Saving them for what?" I asked.

"I like to have a new set in case I have company," she said.

"You're not going to get overnight guests," I said as I continued to open up the package. "Mom, you live in a one bedroom apartment."

"LEAVE THOSE SHEETS ALONE!" she yelled as she grabbed it out of my hand.

"MOM, YOUR SHEETS AND TOWELS ARE FADED

AND THREAD BARE. YOU HAVE NEW ONES SO USE THEM. WHAT ARE YOU WAITING FOR?" I yelled back.

"I'LL USE THEM WHEN I'M GOOD AND READY!" she said.

They were the days that I would get so frustrated trying to reason with Mom. She always felt she needed the security of saving her nice things for the future. This saddened me that my mother felt that she was not worth these simple luxuries.

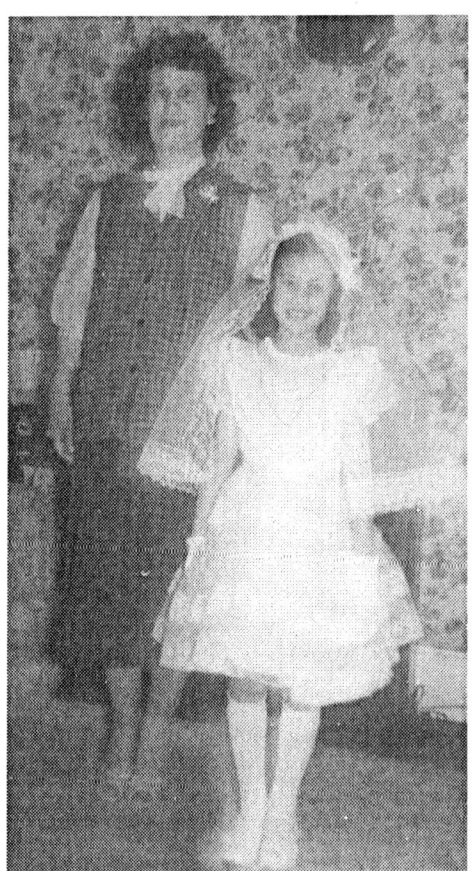

Mom and daughter at First Holy Communion

41
More Memories

Mom seemed to recall more events when we looked at albums from our early days.

"Look Mom, here's a picture of you and me. I'm making my First Holy Communion. And it looks like we're in the house on Moore Street," I said.

"I remember that house. We had flowers," she said as she pointed to the picture of the flowery wallpaper. Sometimes Mom would concentrate on the smallest detail.

"Mom, you look like you're expecting a baby in this picture," I pointed out to her.

Mom was 43-years-old when Chuckie was born. Between my birth and Chuckie's, Mom had two miscarriages, and she was thrilled to finally have her long awaited son. I was way into adulthood when Mom opened up to me about how she learned of Chuckie's condition. She was not told as soon as he was born.

As Mom was taking care of her infant son, she felt that he was not as alert as I had been. During the baby's routine check up, she mentioned this to the physician. The doctor proceeded to tell her that the baby was Mongoloid. At that time, this condition was not discussed. She asked the doctor if there was a cure for this. He told her there was no cure at the present time, but he gave her the name of a specialist to examine the baby. Mom told me she walked home that day with the baby in the stroller somewhat in a daze. Picturing this gave me a lump in my throat.

Gradually Mom started learning more about this condition that caused Chuckie to have severe retardation. The dreams she had for her son were shattered. In 1957, Down Syndrome was not discussed. What a crushing disappointment, especially for someone like Mom who wanted so much for her children.

However, Mom had unconditional love for both of us. For 30 years, she took care of Chuckie at home. This included bathing and dressing him. He seemed to get bronchitis and stomach viruses often, and Mom would stay up most of the night nursing him back to health. She was always very protective towards Chuckie. In those years, I remember Mom praying that she would outlive Chuckie by at least one day so he would always be safe with her. I believe Mom felt somewhat guilty for Chuckie's condition. This caused her to have a lower self-esteem. Mom always worried about Chuckie's future.

My mother and father were older parents when they had him and were realistic about the situation. What a hard decision it was when Mom consented to have Chuckie live in a group home. He was 30 years old, and Mom knew she could not take care of him much longer. She wanted to make sure he had good care and was able to live to his fullest potential.

For Chuckie, the move went smoothly. He adjusted well to his new environment and became more independent. But of course, Mom worried terribly about him. For the longest time, she and Dad picked him up on Wednesdays for dinner. Then they would pick him up every Friday to stay for the weekend. Sunday night Chuckie would go back to the group home. Every holiday and family gathering, Chuckie was included. As it turned out, my brother had the best of both worlds. He still had family life and was able to live semi-independently with a supervisor at the group home. Gradually Mom started feeling comfortable with the situation. Now she still gets to see Chuckie about once a week and in her own way tries to dote on him.

"Mom, here's a picture of you with Grandmom and your brothers and sisters," I said.

She looked and said, "I haven't seen my sister Mary in so long." I just let that comment go. There didn't seem to be a point in telling her that her sister was no longer with us.

Mom's father died when he was 54-years-old leaving behind a wife and eight children. Mom was the third oldest. Now there are only three siblings left. Her older brother, Mike, was killed in a car accident in the early 1940's. Her sister Mary and three of her younger brothers passed away. Now Mom was the oldest in the family with her brother Gus and younger sister Anna.

My grandmother lived with us until she died at 81-years-old. Mom took care of her up to the end. I now marvel at how my mother was able to handle the family and household with the added responsibility of being the only caregiver of my brother and grandmother.

Mom always said, "Maybe that's why the Lord keeps me healthy."

My dad was a long distance truck driver and many times would come home late at night. She would then start cooking all over again and have dinner ready for him. Dad liked his food fried. He seemed to always eat the same thing—fried meat and potatoes. He was too inflexible to try new foods.

I wish that my parents had more fun in their lives. I never remember them going out and cultivating friendships with other couples. I don't even think they ever went to the movies. The few times that they had to go somewhere socially, it seemed to be a big problem. Arrangements had to be made for Chuckie and my grandmother. When there was a family social, Mom would have to bathe and dress Chuckie and my grandmother before she could get ready. Before she even went out, she had to be exhausted.

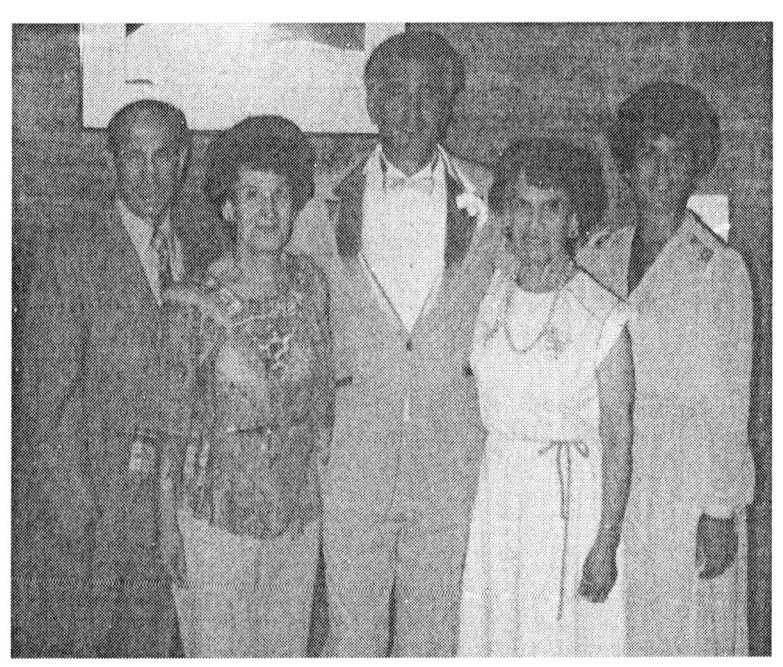

Fran with brothers and sisters

42
Mom Was Always There for Us

I wonder if Mom ever had dreams of romance and adventure. She may have, but I believe Mom's childhood experience of being tormented and feeling so unattractive always stayed with her. Even though she had surgery on her eye so it did not move uncontrollably, she never gained the self-confidence and self worth that she deserved.

For as early as I could remember, Mom conveyed the message that her life was "all about her daughter." That meant my proms, awards in school, and graduation—my dates, social events, and what I was wearing. Mom took so much pride in her daughter. She lived her life vicariously through me. Of course, I didn't need too much convincing that her life should revolve around me. I wasn't any more selfish or self-centered than any other young person, but after all, what else did Mom have to do but serve me.

Those days when I was single and going to work in the morning seemed so long ago. No one in our house ever depended on an alarm clock. Mom was always the first one up in the morning. She needed to get Dad up early for work. Then she would call me. While I was getting dressed, she would bring me a cup of coffee and a piece of toast. When my mother was single, she worked in a pant's factory sewing all day. I never thought my job was that special, but it seemed glamorous to her that I dressed up every morning to go to an air-conditioned office to work as a secretary.

After I left, she would get Chuckie ready for school, and then she would get Grandmom up and organized. While I was at work, if some of us made plans on a spur of a moment to go out that night, I would just call Mom.

"Mom, I'm going out with my friends tonight. I'll come home to change. Could you iron my pink blouse?"

Those days seemed as if I was in a different world.

I know Mom always worried endlessly about me. She wanted so much for me to experience life, but she also wanted to hold me back so I would be protected. I don't think I could ever go out the door without seeing the concerned look on her face saying, "Drive carefully and call me when you get there."

All during my single life I lived with my parents. My mother never went to bed until I was home. A week before I was getting married, Dom and I went to the movies and got a bite to eat afterwards. When Dom took me home that night, of course, Mom was waiting up for me as usual.

"Mom, I'm 23 years old. I'm getting married next week and moving out. Why do you still insist on waiting up for me?" I asked.

"I'm not waiting up for you," she said. "I was just doing a couple things around the house. I didn't realize it got so late," she said.

"Yeah right," I said.

Even after I was married in my own home with my own family, Mom still worried and always wanted to make sure we were all safely home.

43
September 11, 2001

During this time of caregiving for my parents, I really did not pay too much attention to national and world news. That is until 9/11. Along with most people, the events of that day had a big jolt in my thinking. No matter how busy and concerned I was about my family and caregiving, there was a world out there that I took for granted. Mom's mental decline was too far-gone for her to understand the gravity of this situation.

However, Dad was shocked by this disaster. My father was a World War II veteran who fought in four battles overseas to defend his country. Now he watched the news in disbelief as a hijacked passenger jet crashed into the north tower of the World Trade Center. Then a second hijacked airliner crashed into the south tower of the World Trade Center. Both buildings were burning and the streets of New York City were in chaos with people screaming and running. President Bush said that the country has suffered an 'apparent terrorist attack.'

We then continued to learn that an American Airliner crashed into the Pentagon and another airline, also hijacked, crashed near Pittsburgh. We watched the news on the television screen in disbelief, as people were either jumping out of the windows or being thrown from the force of the explosion. The twin towers collapsed leaving a massive cloud of smoke and debris. Dad looked heartsick. We just knew that countless innocent lives were lost. Then my father mustered up his strength and became angry.

"**WHO THE HELL DID THIS?**" Dad wanted to know.

"I don't know Dad, but the reports are pointing to a man named Osama bin Ladin. US Officials feel he is hiding in Afghanistan," I said.

"**Well that Bastard better be hiding good because the United States ain't gonna take this crap,**" he said.

The President addressed the nation that night. His message stated, "These acts shattered steel, but they cannot dent the steel of the American resolve."

I believe Dad was going through a syndrome that was affecting many World War II veterans. Now he has time to think about the war. My father was a decorated soldier who dodged bullets while fighting in battles. He also was the driver of heavy equipment transporting personnel and supplies in black outs.

Many of the WW II servicemen are retired and now have time to think of their military years. I heard some veterans were getting physically and emotionally sick from reminiscing the horror they encountered during a war that took place over half a century ago.

However, I do not think this was the case with my father. He thought quite a lot about his years in the service, but I believe he had a longing to go back to them. Dad associated the days when he served his country as the prime of his life. During that era, he was healthy, strong and productive.

I remember Dad's reaction as we watched President Bush standing in the devastation of the collapsed buildings. The President spoke through a megaphone and stated adamantly that whoever was responsible for this disaster will be hearing from us.

Dad nodded in agreement. "We'll get em," he said. "Hell, I didn't trudge through Europe and watch my buddy get his legs blown off for this," he said. "Now this world isn't safe for Denise and Krissy. I wish I could go and fight again. If only I could."

Most Americans were shocked, frightened, and in need of comfort and assurance that their world will continue. The apartment building where Mom and Dad lived announced that they would be having a support group to talk about this horrific event. I decided to attend with Mom and Dad.

Dad said, "I'm glad Mom doesn't understand what's going on. She would be pretty upset."

At the support group, we said prayers and sang patriotic songs. Different people got up to speak to give comfort and try to alleviate the fear that was permeating throughout the country. I decided to offer my thoughts. I began with trying to find something positive that occurred in spite of this disaster.

A year ago our country went through a bitter presidential race. With that election, it seems as though the country was divided between Democrats and Republicans. This attack brought us back together again. We no longer speak as Democrats or Republicans. We are no longer separated by race or religion. We now stand together as Americans who have been attacked. We have witnessed brave acts of strangers helping one another. Family members seem to forget trivial arguments and are showing their love for each other. Even though our country suffered a bitter attack, we will get through it because when we are united like this, we stand strong.

After my speech, I heard a woman from the audience say, "Amen. There was too much 'me-ism' going around and that hurt this country. Let's get back to basics."

Other people made some comments and offered their thoughts. When this meeting was over, we left feeling a little better mainly because of the connection we had with others who shared the same emotions.

During the weeks that followed this horrific event, people remained shocked and in fear of another disaster occurring.

Sales were down with traveling. Entertainment events were canceled. People were staying home out of fear.

"So the terrorists think they're going to break our economy," Dad said.

"That is part of their plan," I commented. "Everyone has become immobile."

"We can't let these terrorist control our lives," Dad said.

In my caregiving experience, I learned the best way to combat fear was to take some action. I agree with the saying, "If you're not part of the solution, you're part of the problem."

"Instead of sitting here complaining about these terrorists, let's do our patriotic duty," I said.

"What do you think you're gonna do—fight 'em?" Dad said sarcastically.

"YES. We are going to the mall to help our economy. You and Mom both need some new clothes. Let's not be ruled by fear," I stated.

"That's a good idea," Dad agreed. I need a new pair of sneakers," he said. "Let's go."

That day we did our patriotic part in keeping the economy flowing. Mom and Dad got some new clothes and we did not let Osama bin Laden win. Good for us.

Fear was still permeating throughout the country. People were canceling vacations and travel plans. The thought of another disaster was keeping us grounded. I certainly am not a person who takes unnecessary risks.

The day I got home from the shopping trip with my parents, I started to reflect on my family. It occurred to me that I had not seen Kristen in a couple months. She was working as a television anchor in West Virginia. I had an overpowering urge to hug my 24-year-old baby. I didn't think about it too long before I called the airline and bought a ticket to West Virginia for September 26, two weeks after the 9/11 disaster.

"**Are you out of your mind?**" my friend Mary yelled when she heard I was going on a plane.

"Maybe so," I said. "But it might be the safest time to fly with all this security and everyone on guard. Besides I really want to see Kristen."

Arrangements had to be made for my parents. Dom would look in on them, and the veteran's aid would be there two hours a day. I hired another person to come on the weekends. Aunt Anna would be the main caregiver while I was gone.

Before going away, I always wrote clear and concise instructions on white construction paper and placed it in full view on the refrigerator. Each caregiver had a separate poster with her name and set of instructions.

Lillian
Veteran's aid for Dad
Assist in showering and shaving Dad
Linen Closet
Towels and washcloths
Soap and shampoo

Medicine Cabinet in Bathroom
Electric shaver, deodorant, combs, capsules for cleaning teeth,   antiseptics and band-aids

Clean clothes
Top drawer of bureau in bedroom
Undershirts and shorts
Second drawer
Socks and pajamas

Third drawer
Polo shirts and sweaters

Fourth drawer
Sweat pants

Bedroom closet
Robe, button down shirts, and casual slacks

Put dirty clothes in the hamper.

You do not need to fix dinner. My aunt will be coming to give them dinner at 5:00 pm.

Please see that my parents get some exercise. If it is nice weather could you take them outside for a walk? If it is raining, please walk up and down the halls with them. (Need to hold on to them).

Any questions, please notify Ann. Her number is on the side of refrigerator with other emergency numbers.

Medical cards are in the cabinet over the sink. They need the cards if they have to go to the emergency room at Montgomery Hospital.

I will be back Sunday night.

Polly (Weekend)
Drive Mom to hairdresser on Saturday at 11:00 am.
Dad might want to go and wait in the shop with you.

After hairdresser, take them to lunch at Jems
They always order the same meal
Two eggs, home fries, toast and coffee

Take a walk with Mom around the building
(Need to hold on to her)

Before you leave, put finger snacks on the coffee
table for them to munch on.

Sunday
Brunch at Jems

Drive Mom and Dad to visit Chuckie at 2:00 pm
Take the three of them for an ice cream cone
in the area.
Bring Chuckie back to Group Home
Have Mom and Dad back by 5:00 pm

My aunt will take over

Emergency numbers are on the side of refrigerator

Medical cards are in the cabinet over the refrigerator
Montgomery Hospital in an emergency

My aunt will come to give them dinner

Aunt Anna
Mom's clothes are in the armoire
Top drawer
Underwear, socks, nightgowns

Second drawer
Tops and sweaters

Closet
Slacks, robes, jackets

All supplies are in the linen closet for Mom's shower
You could shower her in the morning or evening
(whenever it is more convenient for you)

Remind Mom to brush her teeth in the morning and before bed.

Remind Dad to put his dentures in the cup. You'll have to put in the cleaning capsule.

Sometime during the day, give Dad his eye drops.

Their individual pill compartments are filled for the four days that I will be gone.

The bottles of medications are in the cabinet by the cups. Take all medication with you if they need to be hospitalized.

All-important numbers are on the side of refrigerator including Polly and Lillian.

Also, you could reach me at Kristen's. I will call you to see if everything is going smoothly.

I can't believe I am actually in the plane flying to West Virginia. There were only two other passengers on board with me. The flight attendant changed our seats so there would be more balance in the plane. I pretended that this was my own private aircraft. The flight was uneventful. Thank God. When we landed, one of the passengers looked at me and said, "We made it."

"I guess everyone is a little nervous," I responded.

When I got off the plane, Kristen was waiting for me. What a joy it was to see her. I couldn't stop hugging her. We had a marvelous time together. I went to the TV station and watched all that goes into reporting the news. I was in awe of my daughter.

We went shopping and out to dinner. Then we would stay up late talking at night sharing stories. Kristen was so emotional about 9/11. It was a combination between anger and sadness.

"I just can't believe anyone could commit such a terrible act," she said.

"I know, Honey, it is hard to believe," I agreed.

"Mom, I'm surprised you wanted to fly at this time," Kris said.

"I really wanted to see you, and I wasn't going to let fear of the terrorists stop me," I replied.

"Mom, I feel so sorry for all those kids," she said. "This is horrible."

I looked at Kristen and said, "Yes, we certainly are in a terrible situation. But Kris, it was mostly adults who perished in this disaster. There were very few kids killed."

"But Mom, look at all the kids who now have to grow up without mothers and fathers," she said sadly. "Can you image what their lives are going to be like?"

"You're right. I didn't think about it that way," I said.

Then Kris said, "I cannot imagine growing up without you and Dad."

"Gee Kris, when you were growing up weren't some of the words you used to describe me as strict, manipulative, and a control freak?" I laughed.

"Well you were and still are," she stated. "But when all my girlfriends talk about traits and idiosyncrasies that their mothers have, you don't seem so bad."

"Thanks Kris," I said. "I guess that's suppose to be a compliment," I laughed.

Kristen and I continued to reminisce and share stories throughout the night.

As Kris grows older what mother-daughter memories will she cherish? Will she remember this special time together? Thank God I had so many precious moments with my mother to sustain me.

My visit with Kristen came to an end too quickly, and I was back to my routine. Aunt Anna reported that everything went smoothly.

44
Life Is Still Precious

During this time of constantly rushing and being on the road so much, I got into two car accidents. Fortunately, no one was hurt although my insurance premiums increased. I looked at this as a wake up call for me to slow down and be more careful.

I was too busy to dwell on this whole caregiving situation. But there were times that I felt melancholy because of the loss of our mother-daughter relationship. This emptiness occurred at different times. When I would take Mom for a walk, her language skills had deteriorated so much that it was hard to have a conversation. Her world was now so small that it became an effort to think of things to say. I longed to share my every day happenings with her as I did most of my life. Again, at these moments, I mourned my loss.

However, I learned something from Mom during this stage of Alzheimer's. She lived in the moment. Since we could not enjoy talking about the past or plan for the future, I decided to enjoy the precious moments with her. Now is the only time we have. Most of my life, I have allowed the past and my future concerns to dominate the present moment. Thinking of past mistakes and missed opportunities serves no purpose, and when our minds are always racing to do the next chore, we miss the present moment.

John Lennon once said, "Life is what's happening while we're busy making other plans."

It was a beautiful day that October in 2001. I was driving to the market with Mom. I always cut through Elmwood Park. I noticed the leaves were turning colors. The combination of green, orange, and red was breathtaking. When I was a child, I remember going to this park with Mom. I had not walked there in years. On a spur of the moment, I decided we needed to stroll on these grounds.

"Mom, look how pretty the leaves are," I said. "Would you like to walk here?"

"Okay," she said.

Mom still loved to walk although her coordination greatly declined. She developed a leaning posture and walked with a shuffle. We got out of the car. She was a little unsteady on her feet especially on unfamiliar grounds. Ever since I could remember, Mom grabbed my arm when we crossed the street. Her maternal instinct took over even when I was an adult. Now instead of firmly grabbing Mom to steady her while walking, I just put out my arm and she grabbed it as we strolled.

Together we were able to enjoy the simple pleasure of the leaves crackling under our feet. My mother still had quality to her life. I just had to find it. It started out as an ordinary day, but Mom and I created a precious memory. It was also a learning experience for me to look for the extraordinary in the ordinary.

I was beginning to discover the importance of cherishing each moment instead of always waiting for the event that will change my life. Every instant is equally important in the process of growth—moments that are exciting and beautiful as well as the ones that bring boredom and sadness. When I focused on this fact, ordinary things took on a whole new meaning. Life was precious, and I was grateful.

45
Wandering

The Christmas holidays were approaching. I really did not feel like getting into the festive mood but still pushed myself. I got home from the usual routine with my parents. The aid would be there for the next two hours, but I knew eventually I was going to have to hire more help for the evening. Dad usually was so tired that he would fall asleep in his chair after dinner.

I started rummaging around my loft getting out the Christmas decorations when I received a call from the office of the apartment building where Mom and Dad lived.

"Mrs. DiPaolo, this is Jean from the Jefferson Apartments." Jean was the social worker and coordinator for the residents of the building. I had spoken to her several times on issues regarding my parents.

"There seems to be a problem with your mother," she began tentatively.

"UH OH, what is it?" I asked.

"Apparently your mother decided to walk down the hall from her apartment," Jean said.

"Yeah," I said cautiously.

"Well, I believe your mother got a bit confused," Jean explained. She walked into someone's apartment. Then sat down in their living room."

"Oh No!" I said.

"Well, the woman who lives in that apartment asked her if she needed help to get back to her own place. Your mother replied, 'No, I'm fine.' She isn't making any attempt to leave," Jean said with a concerned tone.

This appalled me. "She never leaves the apartment by herself. Where is my father?" I asked.

"I don't know, but I thought I would call you. Maybe you should come over. Perhaps you could persuade your mother to go back to her apartment," she said.

"I'll be right there," I said.

Most of the people who lived in the building knew that my mother and father were declining in health. The neighbors saw me coming and going with my parents. We would always say hello to them, but Mom and Dad no longer had lengthy conversation with the neighbors.

As I was driving, it occurred to me that Mom seemed to be making a noticeable mental decline during these last couple days. She never wanders out of the apartment by herself. Dad must have fallen asleep as usual on the chair. A frightening thought occurred.

What if Mom wandered out of the building? She could go outside without a coat and wander away. She would freeze to death. Something has to be done.

When I got to the building, Jean greeted me. She said, "We were able to persuade your mother to go back to her apartment. I walked her back."

I felt so embarrassed. I told Jean that I was going to check on Mom. When I went in the apartment, Mom didn't seem to think anything was wrong. She did not even know she wandered in someone else's apartment. I told Dad that he had to make sure she didn't open the door. Mom and Dad were alone in the apartment from 5:00 pm until the next morning when I came to get them ready. That arrangement worked well up until this point. However, they both made a noticeable decline in health. Now, Dad falls asleep shortly after he sits down to watch TV. This past week, Mom's mental capacity seemed to deteriorate to a more advanced level of Alzheimer's disease. I have to think of a new strategy if they are going to stay in the apartment.

I had an idea that I wanted to discuss with Jean. I went back to the office. I told Jean that I really wanted to keep my parents out of the nursing home, but now I needed more help. The people who lived in the Jefferson apartments were all senior citizens, but many of them were in their early sixties and were fairly healthy. I asked Jean if she knew of anyone in the apartment who would like to earn some extra money. All that would be required is to stay with my mother and father for two hours a night from about 6:00 PM to 8:00 PM. The person could sit in the living room and watch television with my parents. Or take my mom for a walk up and down the hallway. That way the night would not be so long for them.

Jean said, "That is a good idea. Your mom and dad should have more stimulation."

Then she offered another suggestion.

"Recently, a volunteer group was started by the residents," she said. "If there is a bad snow storm, these volunteers would check on the people who need more help. I will immediately work on these contacts and set up times in the evening for a volunteer to visit your parents," she said.

I felt a little better. At least there was some plan. Walking in the corridor, I happened to see the lady who lived in the apartment where Mom wandered.

"Is your mother all right?" she asked.

"Yeah, she just got a little confused," I said. "I'm sorry for all this."

The woman said, "Your mother was no problem. I just hope she feels better."

"Thanks for your help," I said.

Now I am not sure if I was more upset about this wandering episode because of the potential danger for Mom or because of my own embarrassment.

Again, I thought, *Life is not fair. Growing up, I was not a wild teenager. I never smoked, drank, or took drugs. I never went to wild parties. I certainly never had any problems that involved police or anyone calling my parents with a bad report. Did I ever embarrass my mother and father?* ***ABSOLUTELY NOT!*** *So why now do I have to contend with this feeling of embarrassment from my parents?* ***LIFE IS CERTAINLY NOT FAIR.***

The behavior of a person with a dementing illness is often very embarrassing to the caregiver. Many families prefer to be very private about their problems, but friends and neighbors usually know something is wrong. In the beginning stages, I would give people a short explanation such as "lately my mother is getting a bit confused." As her illness progressed, I explained to friends or neighbors that my mother was suffering from this debilitating illness. Most people were very helpful and supportive.

46
Time for More Help

The very next day after Mom's wandering experience, I got an identification bracelet with my mother's name, address, and telephone number on it. Mom liked jewelry so she didn't mind wearing this at all times. It is common for people with dementia to wander away from home. There are different reasons for wandering. An impaired individual may simply get lost and then become disoriented trying to find his or her way back home.

Also, if a person with dementia is in a new environment, he or she may decide to wander. This not only presents a threat to the impaired individual but also becomes a challenge to law enforcement who must search for the wanderer. Nearly half of all memory impaired adults who are not located within 24 hours die.

Some victims wander aimlessly through the house from one room to another. This may be a result of restlessness or boredom. Perhaps wandering behavior is a way of communicating the feeling of being lost. Agitated pacing could occur as a result of your loved one feeling upset. During this time, calm your relative by speaking in a reassuring voice. The best solution is to accompany him or her on a refreshing walk, or suggest a task or activity he or she could do.

The Alzheimer's Association has administered a nationwide Safe Return program that provides identification, support, and registration for people suffering with dementia. It provides the impaired individual with an engraved identification bracelet. The person is registered in a national database. This is accessible by law enforcement agencies across the country. Engraved on the back is the wearer's identification number and his or her special medical condition.

Included is a twenty-four hour telephone number that is available to anyone who makes a collect call. Also, the Alzheimer's Association offers training about the Safe Return program to all safety and health personnel. Wearing an ID bracelet could help locate Mom in case she ever wandered away.

Jean called me and said she got three different volunteers to help my parents. Each of the volunteers was assigned a different night to check on my parents. She said they would be glad to walk the halls with Mom so she would get her exercise. One of the volunteers was a couple, Bob and Carol. While Carol walked with Mom, Bob stayed with Dad. To my delight, Bob had an interest in history and enjoyed talking about World War II so they had a lot in common. This seemed to be working, but I knew I was going to have to get more help very soon.

47
December 1, 2001

This Saturday was a nice sunny day. Dom was home from work and decided to put up the Christmas lights outside. I was getting ready to leave to take care of Mom and Dad. I told him I would be back about two in the afternoon.

Today it took awhile to get Mom and Dad organized.

"It's a nice day outside, so we might as well get started on our routine," I said.

On the weekends the veteran's aid did not come so I would have to come back tonight to get their dinner ready. I thought Dad needed a haircut so we first stopped at the barber. While Dad was getting his haircut, Mom and I walked in some of the stores in the strip mall. Mom did not look good. She was pale and walking slowly. We went back for Dad and then decided to get a bite to eat. Maybe that would perk Mom up a bit. I noticed that Mom took a few spoonfuls of her soup and said she didn't want anymore.

"Mom, you hardly ate anything," I said.

"I had enough," she said.

"Well, all right. Are you sure you don't want anymore?" I asked.

Mom nodded to take it away.

Today both my mother and father looked tired. I decided we better not go any place else. So I took them back to the apartment. Dad looked as if he needed his nap. I knew he was going to fall asleep as soon as he sat on the couch. I was afraid Mom would then roam from the apartment. So I decided to let Dad nap without worrying about Mom getting lost. I would take Mom back to my house. She could stay with me for the afternoon. I'll bring her back at dinnertime so she could eat with Dad.

"Mom, why don't you come with me? You could help me with some of my work," I said.

"Okay," she agreed.

When we got to my house, I noticed that Dom had put up all the outside Christmas lights. "Christmas is coming soon Mom. Are you ready for it?" I asked.

She just nodded with an uninterested look.

We sat in the family room. "Mom, how about helping me fold the clothes in this basket," I said.

"Okay," she complied.

Together we folded the clothes. Then I put on the television.

"Mom why don't you watch TV while I prepare something for dinner," I said. "I'll just be right in the kitchen."

Dom came in and was talking to Mom for a little while. Then he came up to me and said, "Mom keeps touching her stomach. Do you think she's alright?" I went to check.

"Mom what's the matter? Does your stomach hurt?" I asked.

"Yeah, I have a little pain here," she said.

"Maybe you should try going to the bathroom," I said.

When Mom came out of the bathroom, I asked, "Do you feel any better?"

"Yeah a little better," she said. Mom seemed restless so I tried to distract her. "Let's look at some pictures," I suggested.

I got out one of the albums, and we started looking at the photos.

"Mom look, here's a picture of me. It looks like I'm expecting a baby," I said.

I remember Mom was so excited and happy to be getting her first grandchild. It was not an easy pregnancy for me. I had a bad case of morning sickness, although it did not confine itself to just the morning. That nauseous feeling occurred all day long for the first trimester. Also, I remember being extremely tired during my pregnancy. Then things started to get a little better. Mom was always trying to push food in me back then. I would go over her house on my lunch break from work, and she would have a nutritional meal ready.

"Make sure you eat," she said. Then in my last trimester, I had to contend with backaches. I couldn't seem to get comfortable. Mom was always hovering over me.

My Aunt Mary commented, "I think your mother wants to go through this for you."

Mom said, "If it were possible, I would. It would be easier than knowing my daughter is suffering through those labor pains."

When her first grandchild was born, Mom was ecstatic. To her delight, Denise was a beautiful baby and so bright. Mom took such pride in her granddaughter. She especially enjoyed taking Denise to the market and going up and down the aisles with Neecee in the cart.

Mom felt so proud when other people commented, "What a beautiful baby!"

I believe Mom was the happiest and most content that I had ever seen her. Her life still revolved around me. Her daughter was happily married to a hardworking man who had a good job. We gave her a beautiful, precocious grandchild. And we just put a deposit down on a lovely home. Our little family was moving forward. As far as Mom was concerned, if I had everything, her life was full.

How time flies, I thought as we continued to look at the photos!

Seven months after I gave birth to Denise, Dom and I started preparing to move into our new home. Around that time one day, I walked into Mom's house with the baby.

"Honey, you're so pale today," she said looking concerned.

"Mom, I don't feel good," I said.

"I can see that. You look terrible," she said. "You're not getting enough sleep. And moving is always hard on a person with all that packing."

"Mom, I think I'm pregnant again," I said.

Mom just rolled her eyes in disbelief.

"How could this be? You're not even healed yet from giving birth. And you're still breastfeeding," she said.

"I know," I cried.

"I didn't think you could get pregnant while breastfeeding," she said.

"Well, I don't think it's completely impossible," I said.

Mom said, "But I remember years ago hearing woman say they would nurse for two years so they wouldn't get pregnant. Grandmom breast fed all of us and we're all two years apart."

"I guess it worked for everybody but me," I cried.

Mom let out a long sigh.

"Maybe you're just run-down. Or you could have a virus," she said.

"I doubt it," I cried. At that point, I felt a wave of nausea come over me, so I ran to the bathroom. Mom followed me and held my head as I violently threw up.

"When you're throwing up, I told you always to kneel down," she said. "It takes the pressure off you." Then Mom got a cool washcloth to put on my neck.

"Mom, take care of the baby," I said. "I need to rest for a few minutes."

"I'll get Neecee and you go lay down and rest," she said.

Mom kept my bedroom looking the same as when I lived there. It was comforting to lie on my bed. Mom then came in holding Denise and sat on the bed.

"Feeling any better?" she asked with her worried look.

I nodded.

Then Mom handed me some crackers. "I can't eat anything," I said.

"Try forcing them down. Remember how it was the last time. You'll feel better if you eat little meals often," she insisted.

I complied and forced down two crackers.

"Mom, what am I going to do? I can't go through this again. How am I going to take care of Denise while I'm vomiting all day long? And I'm so tired," I cried.

At that point, Denise decided she wanted some attention. She wanted her mommy to hold her. While I was lying down, I held out my arms and she squirmed all over me.

"Cille, be careful. Don't let the baby sit on your stomach," Mom scolded. "Make her lie down beside you." Then she put a rattle in Neecee's hand to occupy her.

"Did you make a doctor's appointment?" Mom asked.

I nodded, "Yeah, Wednesday."

"The most important thing now is for you to take care of yourself. Did you completely stop breastfeeding Neecee?" she asked.

I nodded yes again.

"Well that's good. This new baby needs to get all the nutrition from you," she said. "Eat more of these crackers before you start feeling queasy again," Mom insisted.

I ate another one slowly.

"Well," Mom said as she sighed again, "you would probably want another baby eventually. So now it's going to be a little sooner than expected."

"I just dread going through this again," I cried.

"Why don't you try taking a nap for a little while? I'll take care of Neecee," she suggested.

"Okay," I agreed. "There's baby food and juice in my bag. And diapers," I said.

"Don't worry, you just rest. We'll be fine," Mom said.

It did feel good to take a nap without worrying about Denise. After my nap, I felt a little better. Before I got up from my bed,

Mom came in with these little baked potatoes. "Eat these," she insisted. "Remember last time, baked potatoes helped stop that nauseous feeling."

I started to eat but could only eat one.

"I guess I better start home before traffic gets heavy," I said as I got up slowly.

"I'll help you get the baby in the car. Then I might as well stay outside to wait for the bus to bring Chuckie home," she said. "Take the rest of these potatoes home to snack on," Mom said as she wrapped them in foil.

We got the baby situated in the car, and as usual, Mom went through her ritual.

"Be careful driving."

"Don't let the baby distract you. If you feel like you're going to vomit, pull over to the side of the road and stop."

"I know Ma. I know Ma," I said with a bit of exasperation.

"OH! YOU KNOW, YOU KNOW!" Mom retorted. "Well, it's pretty obvious, you don't know as much as you think you know. Make sure you eat those potatoes before you feel sick," she said. I started laughing at that point. As I pulled out of the driveway, Mom yelled out, "Call me when you get home."

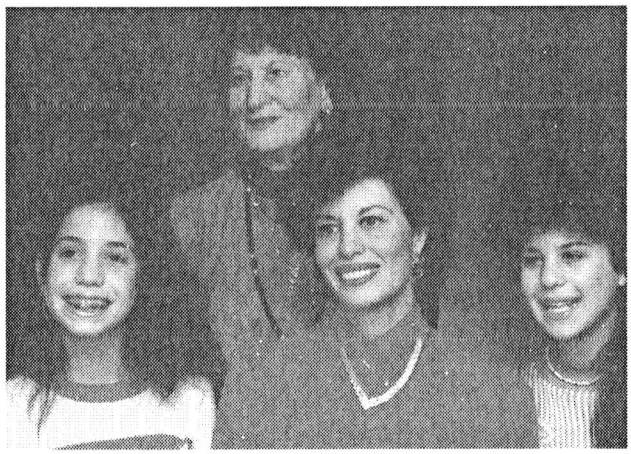

Three Generations

48
A Flood of Memories

It was another very difficult pregnancy. Again Mom hovered over me holding my head through vomiting and dry heaves. Or she was pushing food on me.

"One thing about the women in our family," Mom said, "we have no problem getting pregnant. But The Blessed Mother knows—What we go through to have a baby!"

I remember the day I was in the hospital after giving birth to another baby girl. Mom came in the room. She looked a bit surprised and worried at my appearance.

"What are they doing to you?" Mom asked with her concerned tone.

"I had to be catheterized," I said.

"You look so pale and exhausted," Mom said.

I just shrugged my shoulders. "Did you see my little Krissy yet?" I asked.

"Yeah, but she's not so little. Krissy looks like a strong, healthy baby," Mom said as she was beaming. "So you have two beautiful daughters, Thank God." Then she said in an admonishing tone, "I hope you don't do this again. Those two babies need a healthy mother. Cille, you are going to have to start taking better care of yourself. And besides, I cannot go through this again," she stated adamantly.

Fortunately, Krissy was a very content baby. But it was hard having two babies fifteen months apart. Denise still took a bottle while Krissy was being breastfed. Both were in diapers. For the next three years, I rarely got an uninterrupted night's sleep. My immune system was depleted. I always had a cold or virus. I lost so much weight and was extremely anxious. I also felt angry with myself. I had everything I ever wanted, but I did not think I was handling it well. This brought on guilt. The only person I could truly confide in without feeling I would be condemned was Mom.

"Mom, it is so hard to keep everything together. I'm just going all day but not accomplishing anything."

"Honey, you want everything to be too perfect, and it just can't be that way," she said. "You have to ease up on yourself."

"But it seems other people can handle life without getting so frustrated," I said.

"You don't know what really goes on in other people's lives," she said. "I could see how your life could be so overwhelming."

"I know your life was hard, Mom," I said, "and you seemed to get through it."

"And you'll get through it too," Mom stated.

"I guess," I sighed.

"You know, Cille, in a lot of ways, I had it much easier than you," Mom said trying to restore my confidence. "Remember, I had Grandmom living with us. If I ran out of bread or milk, I didn't have to bundle two babies up and put them in car seats and drive to the market. I was able to just walk out of the house to the corner store or butcher and get what I needed. And you're always trying to be super mom taking the babies to swimming and gym lessons. That has to be exhausting. I never did that. Kids played outside." Mom continued, "And just be content for now that your house can't always look like a picture in a magazine."

In those days just having Mom to call and unload my feelings was a tremendous help.

After about five years of this stage, things started to feel better. Denise was in kindergarten and Krissy was in nursery school. With my free mornings, I decided I was going to take a course in college. I would leave after the girls went to school and would be home in time for them.

That was another big thrill in Mom's life—her daughter going to college. I loved being a student. Eventually I took two courses each semester. Mom just thought it was the neatest thing that her daughter was a mother of two and a college student.

Looking at these pictures brought on another memory that occurred during this time. A new neighbor just moved in the house next door to me. They were a lovely couple with two little boys. For the first couple weeks, we both just said a friendly hello as we saw each other. One day I struck up a conversation with Cathy and got to know so much about her. I learned that Cathy and her husband were renting the house. She told me they still had their house in New Jersey but her mother lived around here. Cathy explained that her mom was going to undergo open-heart surgery.

Being a nurse, Cathy felt if she lived close to her mother, she could give her the care during the months that followed the surgery. Cathy looked extremely anxious and tired. As I got to know her better, I learned she had the same feelings and doubts that I had just a few years ago. I sensed that she needed a friend.

"Why don't you come in for a cup of coffee," I said. "That way we could sit and talk before the kids start coming home." As we sat in my kitchen sipping our coffee, Cathy began opening up to me.

"I just go and go all day, but I never seem to catch up," she said.

"I know how you feel," I empathized. "And I bet when you are running to doctors with your mother, you're feeling guilty because your children aren't getting your attention."

"Exactly," she said. "And we have to pay the mortgage on our house in New Jersey besides the rent here. It is a fortune. I'm just grateful that my husband agreed to do this," she said.

"Well Cathy, that's probably another thing you feel guilty about," I sympathized.

"You got that right. Cille, I get so angry at myself sometimes for not being able to handle this," she confided.

"I know the feeling. I've been there. I remember how easy it is to lose self-confidence," I said.

Cathy looked at me with a surprised expression.

"But you look so together. I envy you when I see you getting into your car with your books going off to school. I wish I could do that," she said.

"Well Cathy, I think everyone goes through bad periods in their lives. A couple years ago, I felt just the way you do. I can see you are really overloaded with responsibility," I said.

"I can't believe you know exactly how I feel," she said.

Then I found myself giving Cathy the same pep talk that Mom gave me when I needed reassurance.

"Cathy believe me, this is a hard time for you, but it will pass." I said. "And I think you are doing a great job. But the only person you're not being good to is yourself."

Cathy nodded, "Thanks for saying that. I feel a little better now," she said.

"Listen Cathy, whenever you're feeling like life is getting too much and you need to talk to someone, just knock on my door. I really think you are doing a great job, but you need to believe it," I said.

"Thanks again, especially for understanding," she said.

When Cathy left that day, I remember thinking how lucky I was to have a healthy mother. There were times throughout my life that I had wished Mom was younger and more with the modern times. However, up until the last few years, Mom was always there when I needed her. Mom was right when she said that you really do not know what another person is going through.

As I sat here on the sofa next to Mom, I wondered how Cathy was doing. It is odd that I am thinking of her at this time. We only had a brief friendship. When she moved away, we did not stay in touch.

"Look Mom, here are the pictures of my graduation," I said as we continued to look at the album. "Do you remember how excited you were?"

Mom nodded yes, but I doubt that she remembered. I recall her keeping some of these pictures in her pocketbook for the longest time. She loved showing them to her friends— especially the one of me in my cap and gown standing in the middle of my two daughters.

In five more months, Denise will be graduating from medical school. What a thrill it would be for Mom if she could only understand this event! That beautiful, precocious baby that Mom loved to be seen with at the market will become Dr. Denise Michelle DiPaolo. I guess this event is coming a little too late for Mom to enjoy.

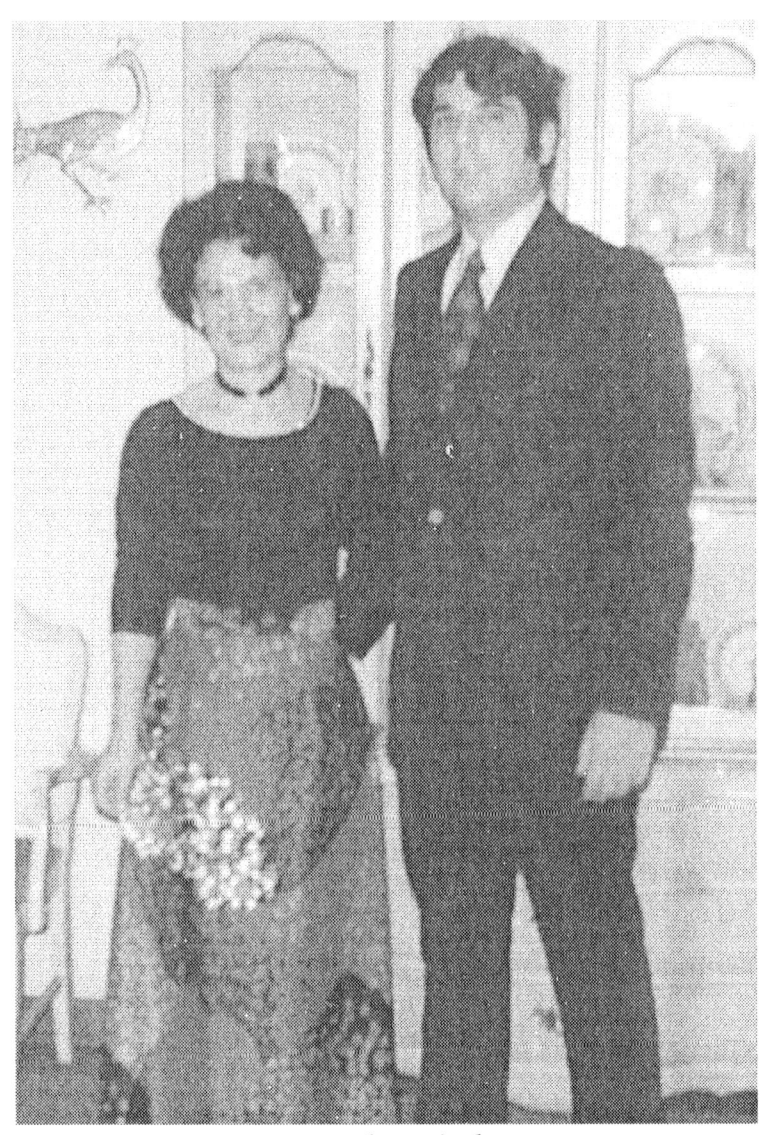

Mom and son-in-law

49
Mom Seemed Restless

Mom seemed uncomfortable sitting here today. "Does your stomach still hurt, Mom?" I asked.

"Yeah, I wonder if the pain will ever go away," she said with a worried look.

"Of course it will," I said. "I get pains all the time. And they always go away. We'll wait a little while, and if your stomach still hurts, we'll go to the doctor."

Then Dom said, "Maybe Mom should stay with us tonight if she isn't feeling well."

"That's probably a good idea," I said, "but I'm still going to have to go back to the apartment and bring Dad his dinner."

"How about if I go and check on Dad, and you stay here with Mom?" Dom said.

"That's a good idea," I said, "and when you're at the apartment, could you get some of Mom's clothes and toothbrush?"

"Okay," he said. "I'll be back in about two hours."

"Just make sure Dad takes his pills," I said. "You have to actually put them in his hand with a glass of water and watch him. Otherwise he won't take them."

"Don't worry," Dom said as he smiled. "I know. Call me if you need me."

"Are you hungry, Mom?" I asked.

"No," she said.

"Are you sure? Maybe that's what is causing your stomach ache," I said.

"My stomach doesn't hurt anymore," Mom said.

"Oh that's good," I said feeling a bit relieved.

"Want to look at more pictures, Mom?" I asked.

"Yeah, there's a lot of them here," she noticed.

"Look Mom, here's a picture of you holding Krissy." Mom glanced at the photo. "You used to call her 'Sugar Plum Krissy.'" Mom smiled. That may have sparked a memory.

Mom would be so proud of Kristen today. Kristen graduated from Syracuse University in 1999 as a broadcast journalist. At that time, Mom's mental capacity was noticeably declining. Kristen now works as a television news anchor in West Virginia. If Mom knew that her sweet little 'Sugar Plum' was a news reporter on television, she would be ecstatic. I had to smile as I pictured Kristen growing up with her sense of adventure. This sometimes caused her grandmother to feel somewhat distressed.

Mom would say, "Why does Kristen have to go so far away to college?"

I explained to Mom, "The girls seem to want the whole college experience."

"I don't understand that," Mom complained. "They both have a nice bedroom and bathroom. They get a home cooked meal. So why would they want to live in a crowded dormitory and eat food from an institution? It seems crazy to me," she stated with exasperation.

I would never be able to make Mom understand so I just shrugged my shoulders and said, "Well if they don't like it, they could always come home."

When Kristen was in her junior year at college, she spent a semester at the Syracuse University campus in London. Mom was appalled. She never heard of such a thing.

"It's bad enough that Kristen has to be so far away from home for college. But going to another country. This seems ridiculous," Mom flatly stated.

"Well, these days lots of the kids go to other countries to study for a semester," I explained. "It's part of the cultural experience."

"CULTURAL EXPERIENCE! IT'S A BUNCH OF BULL!" Mom insisted.

All during the time that Kristen was out of the country, Mom kept asking, "When is 'My Krissy' coming home? Isn't the semester over yet?"

Actually the semester was over, but there was no sense telling Mom that Kristen and a couple girlfriends were backpacking through Europe.

50
Imagine How Mom Feels

I continued to sit with Mom trying to figure out how to relieve her stomachache. If only Mom could explain exactly how she feels. I don't know if she is constipated or maybe she has a bladder infection. Could she be coming down with a virus? What should I do?

Then I imagined what life must be like for anyone suffering from Alzheimer's. I looked at the stack of albums. Those books represented a lifetime of my memories. Older portraits were in black and white, and as technology advanced, the pictures show the beautiful colors. The albums represented my life—places I have been, people I love, and the good times we shared. Each photo sparked more recollections. Some were happy and exciting; others brought memories of uncertainty and sadness. Those memories sum up my life's experience and give meaning to my existence. They determine who I am and how I think. They will shape the decisions I will make in the future. My memory is my identity that holds my life together.

What a frightening thought to look at these photos and be unable to recognize the people or recall any of these events. I would not be able to reminisce with my cousin Stefanie about our traditional Christmas Eve celebration at our grandmother's house when we were kids.

There would be no recollection of my lifetime friend Theresa and how we would go trick or treating until our big pillowcases were filled with candy. And I would never remember when my friend Connie and I went down the shore and came home with a bad case of sunburn. That was a definite learning experience.

There were all these memories with Dom—our first date, the movie, *Camelot*, falling in love, and our life together with our daughters. Without a memory, all these people would be strangers, and my past life would be gone. I would no longer be able to relive these events in my mind. It would be as if my life never happened.

Then I thought of how confused and frightened Mom must have felt as her memory gradually slipped away. What a lonely existence not to remember her life. She lost her identity. Mom had no connection with her past, present, and future. In losing her memory, a big part of her life was gone.

Yet, I still felt there was some quality to Mom's life. She still enjoyed food and was able to feed herself. Also, she remained continent, which was a big plus, and it made it possible for me to be her caregiver. She liked the outdoors and was able to walk, although I noticed her coordination greatly declined. I wondered what was to come. I know there was no place to go but down. Would I eventually have to watch my mother become completely bedridden and lose control over bodily functions? Thinking of Mom deteriorating to this vegetative state was frightening.

51
Going to the Hospital

Mom was getting restless again and looked uncomfortable. Then I noticed her stomach seemed slightly distended.

I said, "Mom, it looks like your pants are too tight. Maybe that's why your stomach hurts."

"Oh, for heaven sakes," Mom said with a bit of embarrassment.

"Let's undo the top button. That will give you some breathing room," I said.

We both started laughing at such a simple solution. However, I felt something was seriously wrong. This morning when I helped Mom get dressed, the slacks were not tight over her stomach.

"Mom, lie down on the couch for a little while," I suggested. Mom complied.

Her protruding stomach was definitely not normal. My thought was that Mom had a urinary tract infection and was not able to completely pass her water. I know that feeling is uncomfortable. So I decided to take Mom to the emergency room at the hospital. They could catheterize her, which would give her some relief. In the meantime, Dom came home from taking care of Dad.

As Dom was coming in he said, "Dad ate dinner, took his

pills and then I helped him get ready for bed. I told him Mom wasn't feeling well so she is going to stay with us tonight."

"Does Dad seem okay?" I asked.

"Just a little tired. He said you wore him out today at the shopping center."

Then I told Dom what I thought was wrong with Mom, and I was going to take her to the emergency room. Mom's stomach was looking worse now, and she seemed to be in pain. Dom suggested, "Instead of driving, let's call an ambulance."

I thought that was a better idea, so I called 911.

"Mom, we are going to get you some help for this stomach ache," I said. "The doctor will be able to help you at the hospital."

"Okay," she said as she lay on the couch.

The paramedics came and got her on the stretcher. I stayed with Mom reassuring her that I would be right by her side so she would not feel confused and afraid. I rode in the ambulance, and Dom followed in the car.

As I sat in the ambulance listening to the siren, I wondered if this was real. It was odd but on the way to the hospital, I remembered my mother telling me about the first time she ever rode in an ambulance. It was in 1971 when Mom was taking care of her mother. My grandmother was afraid of hospitals and never wanted to go. Mom took care of her up until her last few days. Then she felt my grandmother would be more comfortable with the technology and equipment at the hospital. But Mom did not leave her side. She told me that it felt unreal when she was riding in that ambulance with her mother. And now 30 years later, I am having that same feeling.

When we arrived at the emergency room, I told the doctor that I suspected a urinary tract infection. The doctor examined Mom, but he suspected something different—an abdominal aneurysm. Mom was given x-rays. When the x-rays came back, it was confirmed. She had an aneurysm that was internally bleeding. The prognosis was bleak. Mom was given painkillers so her stomach ache was relieved. The nurse came in and said, "Mrs. Engro, your room is ready. We can wheel you upstairs now."

"You mean I have to stay here tonight," Mom said as she looked at me. "I feel good now. I can go home."

"Mom, it's best to stay for the night to make sure your stomach ache doesn't come back," I said.

We got up to the room. I could tell the drugs were starting to make her sleepy. I talked to the attending nurse, and she assured me that Mom would be comfortable. If the pain returned, Mom would be given more medication.

Mom looked very content as I sat by her bedside. "Mom, do you need anything?" I asked.

"No," she said.

"How does your stomach feel? Do you still have that pain?" I asked.

"No I don't have any pain," she said.

"That's good," I said. I thought it was odd. Mom sounded more coherent than she had in a long time.

"Do you want me to stay here with you?" I asked.

"No, I'm fine. You better go home. I want to go to sleep," Mom said.

"Well, okay. We'll both get a good night's rest, and I'll be back for you tomorrow," I said. "Sleep tight Mom as I bent down to kiss her forehead. I love you."

"I love you too," she said as she closed her eyes.

52
December 2, 2001

Dom and I left the hospital about 11:30 pm. By the time we drove home and got into bed, it was way after midnight. It was a long day. I was just dozing off when the phone rang. Not fully alert, I picked up the receiver and said hello. The person on the other end of the phone was telling me my mother died peacefully in her sleep.

For the next fifteen minutes, I just laid in bed trying to mentally digest this phone call. Then I said the words out loud. "My mother is dead."

Then I said the words as a question. "My mother is dead?" "My mother is dead?"

How could that be? She was just walking around and shopping with me? I have to see her. Why didn't we stay at the hospital? I knew an aneurysm was serious, but I assumed she would linger. We went back to the hospital. Mom was still lying in the hospital room. She looked peaceful. I had to touch her face and hand to be sure she really was dead. My feelings were part disbelief. My mother was really gone. Also, I felt relieved that Mom died a merciful death.

For three and a half years, I watched my mother's mental state decline. However, I believe she was lucky. Mom was able to maintain quality to her life and had a dignified death.

I do not know how much longer she could have maintained this condition. Now I would not have to go through the devastating pain of watching my mother deteriorate to existing in a vegetative state.

So much had to be done. I went through the next few days preparing for the funeral. The adrenaline must have kicked in because I missed a whole night sleep, but I had unusual energy to get everything done. That was something that surprised me because normally when I do not get enough sleep, I feel lethargic and sometimes in a fog. I was able to make all arrangements. Also, my dad needed a great deal of help. He was distraught. I was worried about him making it through the next few days.

Dad looked dazed as he said, "I was the one who was suppose to go first. She went for a walk and never came back."

"Dad, maybe you shouldn't go to the funeral. It's going to be a long day. I'm not sure you have the energy," I said.

He said adamantly, "No, I want to be there."

53
My Final Good-Bye

For my final good-bye to my mother, I wrote the eulogy written as a letter from me to Mom. I asked my cousin Anita to read this on my behalf at the graveside.

Dear Mom,

From the time you brought me into the world, we shared an extremely close mother-daughter bond. You were always a big part of my life. Now, I can be comforted with beautiful memories that I will always cherish.

My most precious memories of us are the things that occurred on ordinary days. When I drive through Main Street, I remember being a little girl shopping with you and getting a hot dog at Woolworth's. As we crossed the street, you automatically would grab my arm, a habit that you had even when I became an adult. I remember the homemade pizza that we just couldn't stop eating and your connolis at Christmas.

As I grew older, our bond grew stronger. You were not only my mother but also best friend and confidante. You shared my joys and comforted me through my disappointments. You also had the special gift to hold me close and at the same time, let me go. I'm going to miss that comforting smell of coffee as I walk through your door. And when it starts to rain or snow, I am going to miss hearing that phone ring and just knowing that's my mom checking to see if I'm safely home.

I believe everyone has a purpose in life, and we may all wonder sometimes what our special purpose is and whether we are fulfilling it. When I think of what your life was about, it is easy to see a nurturer. You had an extraordinary energy for the people you loved. We relied on your inner strength and quiet courage that you used every day of your life. You always put the needs of your family first. The patience you showed while caring for your own mother was endless. In the last couple months, we talked of Grandmom, and you were comforted by feeling that you had your own special angel watching over you. You were devoted to Dad for 53 years. And you were the most loving and caring mother to Chuckie and me. What a role model I had!

When I became a mother, your love and concern extended to your precious granddaughters. I remember the joy we shared when Denise was born. How proud you were. You loved hearing about our accomplishments. But you also worried a lot. You were always concerned that Denise was working too hard. When Kristen was living in other countries, you were always asking, "When is Krissy coming home?"

In the last few years as you gradually slipped away, we had to switch roles. Even then, you wanted to protect me. You were concerned that you were causing me too much work and would say, "Leave it go, I'll do it later." And Chuckie was constantly on your mind. I believe the Lord gave you a special son because he needed an extraordinary mother. In the last few days, you talked of your brother Gus who was always so precious to you. I would always assure you that Uncle Gus was loved and cared for by his devoted family.

Most of your life was spent in good health and for this you were grateful to God. Now that we must part, I will treasure the years we spent together. I get a sense of comfort in thinking of your passing as finishing your job and you could go Home. Now, I have my own special angel watching over me. So until we meet again Mom, I love you with all my heart. I feel very fortunate to be your daughter.

Love,
Lucille

Then I helped Dad and Chuckie place their flowers on the casket. I placed mine and said "Good-bye Mom. I love you."

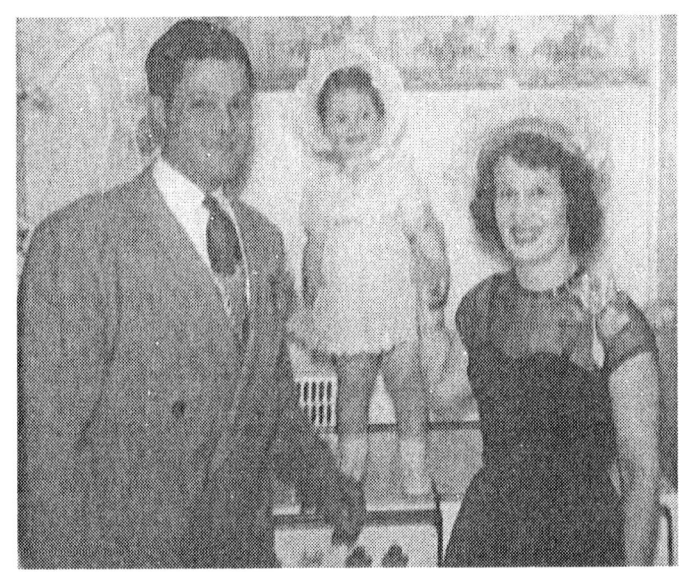

Dad, Lucille, Mom

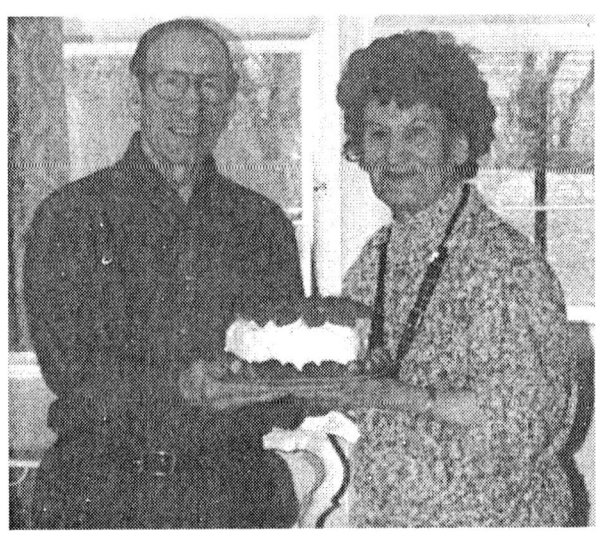

Fran and brother, Gus

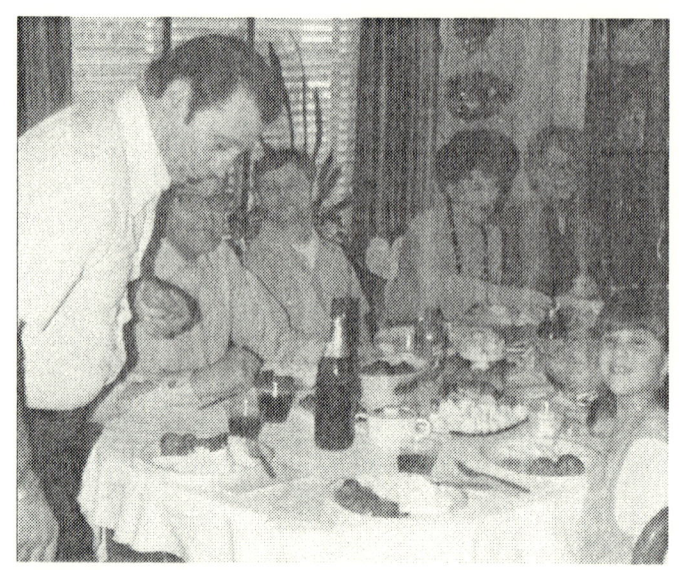

Mom with family at table

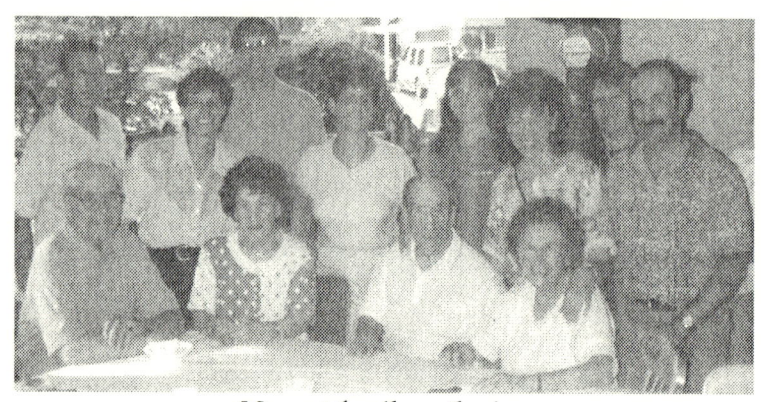

Mom at family gathering

54
Meaningful Accomplishment

The growth and learning experience from dealing with my mother's affliction with Alzheimer's disease has been one of my most meaningful accomplishments. Before I was the primary caregiver of my parents, I would have defined my significant accomplishments with the external aspects of life—buying a home, getting a degree, or making money. These goals are necessary to improve my circumstances in life and undoubtedly, still give me pleasure. However, the elation I feel from these achievements is short lived. Then I reach for another asset. Learning about Alzheimer's disease through my mother's affliction caused me to redefine my priorities.

I now think of my most meaningful accomplishments as realizing my internal capacity. As I watched dementia rob my mother of her memory, I gained a strength that I did not know existed within me. In the three and a half years of her illness, I learned to stay centered through disasters. I learned to deal with my negative emotions such as anger, frustration, guilt, and depression.

Acknowledging my fears was a step forward in my growth. When a new situation arises, I stop worrying about making mistakes. I find it is best to jump in and do the tasks as best I can. Also, I mastered tackling problems by taking things in manageable portions. Not all decisions must be made at one time. Sometimes getting through each day is enough of an accomplishment.

As these daily challenges occurred, I found the value in love, understanding, and empathy. In the midst of adversity, I discovered one of the best coping tactics is a sense of humor. Some days I was quite proud of myself for enhancing my creativity while dealing with my mother's personality changes.

I asserted myself to seek and accept help. The job of caregiving is too big for one person without feeling isolated, which creates more stress. I have become conscientious about taking care of my own health. Everyone is vulnerable to illness. I learned to accept change. Nothing ever stays the same.

When I thought of being a caregiver as a growing opportunity, I received a wealth of knowledge through reading books, learning from others, and my own personal experience. I gained self-confidence and apply what I learned in these years to other situations in life.

Throughout this part of life's journey, the final lesson Mom taught me is to be aware of time moving forward. Do not hold on to the past so tightly. Be ready to come into the present. Live each precious moment to the fullest. I am grateful for this experience and all that I have discovered about myself. I truly believe that dealing with Alzheimer's disease through my mother's illness is one of my most meaningful accomplishments.

55
Advocates Needed

In the past, when there has been a major health problem affecting a huge portion of people, Americans have always responded with demands in more government funding for research and improved health care. Despite the staggering human and financial costs of this brain-wasting illness, Alzheimer's still does not have a high enough profile for the government to increase significant funding for care, treatment, and prevention of this disease. Perhaps it is because people suffering from dementia are seldom able to speak for themselves. They do not organize public demonstrations or lobby elected officials to express dissatisfaction over government funding. The family members who are directly involved in the care of a loved one are much too busy to participate in a political movement. Therefore, it becomes easy to ignore the elderly in our society.

Organizations such as The Alzheimer's Association and Alzheimer's Disease and Related Disorders Association have been effective in increasing awareness and raising federal allocations for research in Alzheimer's. However, in comparison to funds for other public health problems, the Alzheimer's disease research expenditures fall short.

Robert N. Butler MD, founding director of the National Institute on Aging has cautioned, "We remain ill-prepared for the twenty-first century when population aging will become unprecedented...I regard the baby boomers as a generation at risk."[35]

Being part of the health conscious baby boomer generation, I am concerned since we will make up a huge part of the elderly population. In the USA, it is estimated that over four million Americans already suffer from Alzheimer's and 360,000 will be added each year. American businesses lose approximately $61 billion a year due to time lost at work by caregiver's turnover and replacement training. Alzheimer's is costing our country $100 billion dollars annually according to the estimates used by the Alzheimer's Association.[36] Most of this is privately paid, but the costs to the government and businesses are already huge and will continue to grow as the number of people with Alzheimer's increases.

The incidence of Alzheimer's disease doubles every five years among people over 65.[37] Today it is estimated that 35 million Americans are 65 or older. As the baby boomers reach age 65 in fewer than 10 years, the number of workers relative to retirees will decline. By 2030, our entire baby boomer generation will be over 65. The number of Americans with Alzheimer's will soar. The combination of the aging population and the financial costs of this illness will be devastating.

Hillary Rodham Clinton refers to the old African adage "It takes a village to raise a child." Groups have criticized her for trying to put the responsibility of the parents on the government.

The former First Lady responded by saying, "The task of child rearing is so crucial to society that it needs to be seen as both a personal and collective endeavor."

This same argument could be applied to the responsibility of caring for people with Alzheimer's. This disease will take a heavy toll on society. In the next several decades, we will pay either directly or indirectly.

The main purpose of biomedical research is to prevent the disease. Although there has been some progress, this is still a dream and may take many more decades to see dramatic results. In the meantime, there must be increased attention given to helping those who currently suffer from Alzheimer's. The quality of life depends more on human compassion and skill than on medical breakthroughs. This also requires increased funding.

Families need easy access to affordable training, education, and counseling programs.

Companies need to develop eldercare assistance programs, enabling employees to use sick and family leave for the care of a disabled parent.

A family member who provides much of the caregiving should receive a tax credit. They are providing a financial saving to society.

Long-term care needs to be addressed by Medicare and Medicaid. They need to pay part of the prescription drugs and services such as adult day care, home care, and respite care.

Government incentives need to be developed for alternatives to nursing home care.

The ultimate goal of preventing Alzheimer's disease will be realized when a critical mass of people decides that this is a priority worth funding on a large scale. Also, the goal of improving the life of individuals already affected requires funding. Advocates are needed to raise money and pressure elected officials into allocating a bigger portion of government funds. The Alzheimer's Association is the leading organization in the United States in this advocacy effort. The association is seeking to increase funds to $1.4 billion annually for researching ways to prevent and treat this brain wasting disease. Also representatives are seeking a tax credit up to $3,000 to assist the family caregivers in the costs of home and day care for their afflicted loved ones.[38]

This debilitating illness is not just a problem confined to the United States. On June 20, 2005, the first estimate of the worldwide costs of dementia care was released at the Alzheimer's Association International Conference on Prevention of Dementia. The worldwide cost of this disease is estimated at $156 billion. As a result of this staggering amount, advocates are calling for increased funding in research to eliminate Alzheimer's disease.

William Theis, Ph.D., vice president of the Alzheimer's Association of Medical and Scientific Affairs stated, "Our choice is now clearer than ever. Either increase funding for Alzheimer's disease research...or sit back and wait for it to overwhelm the health systems in the U.S and throughout the world."[39]

56
Hope for the Future

People with Alzheimer's disease have problems with short-term memory. They have trouble remembering details about the present or recent past. They may wonder if they paid that bill or took their medication? Many of us have a problem forgetting at times, but older people are particularly susceptible to lapses in recent memory.

However, a lapse in memory may not always be a sign of Alzheimer's or a brain disorder. Sometimes forgetfulness is caused by fatigue or poor physical health.

When Alzheimer's disease is present, a mild memory loss does not stay the same over a period of years. It progresses from occasional forgetfulness to a more serious form of mental confusion. During this progression, the personality of the victim can change. The person can show agitation, hostility, and paranoia.

Society should **never** accept this deterioration of the mind as a normal part of aging. A confused state should not be considered the natural consequence of growing old. These are symptoms of an illness. If we recognize that memory impairment in the elderly is a disease, we have hope for the future. A disease is an illness that could be treated and cured.

Many experts believe that ongoing research will determine the benefits of cardiovascular health in its relationship to dementia. A strategy to delay the onset of Alzheimer's by five years could reduce the number of people affected by one half over the next 50 years. When the cause of this brain-wasting illness is discovered and an effective treatment is developed, the elderly population will be able to spend their remaining years mentally alert and productive.

President John F. Kennedy said, "It is not enough for a great nation merely to have added new years to life. Our objective must also be to add new life to those years."

57
My Memory Booster

After being a caregiver for my parents, I have become very aware of my own memory or sometimes lack of it.

How could I have forgotten that appointment? Did I pay that bill? What's that person's name?

Yet some people marvel at how I could remember the social security numbers of my whole family. It seems that many of my friends are experiencing similar episodes with their memories.

There is no one answer for enhancing memory, but I am aware of one of the culprits. Multitasking—it has become an accepted way of life. In my observation, I rarely find a person only doing one thing at a time. New technology is supposed to make our lives more effective but it has an opposite effect. Cell and cordless phones make it possible to converse while cooking, cleaning, or grocery shopping. I remember being in a restaurant when a pager went off. Three people including my husband looked to see if it was for them.

I have found an interesting pastime of people watching when I am a passenger in a car. To my amazement, drivers get very creative while at the wheel. I have come to the conclusion that no one just drives anymore. The task of operating an automobile is combined with talking on the phone, shaving, dental flossing, and applying make-up.

Another observation is our vehicle has taken the place of the dining room table for mealtime. Have you ever noticed how many people eat while in the car? Just look at the drive-in lines at the fast food places.

Why is it that we can't get into a car even for a short drive without a beverage? When did our nation get so thirsty? Let me test my memory. Was it when the manufacturer's started making cars with cupholders? Oh the power of suggestion!

I am not condemning anyone for this, especially since I am just as guilty. But living in this frenzied society is craziness disguised as multitasking. Is it any wonder that we cannot remember what we had for lunch?

When we do too many things at one time, it is impossible to concentrate and remain focused. We become less effective and lose much of our enjoyment in the activity. We automatically do so many tasks simultaneously that it never registers in our brains as a vivid memory.

In looking for ways to improve my memory, I tried my own experiment. I block out one hour each day when I commit to doing one task at a time. If I am doing something mundane such as ironing or washing dishes, I try focusing just on that activity for the hour. If I am talking on the phone, I completely focus on the conversation.

To my delight, I have noticed several changes. I have become more interested in the activity that I am performing. Also, the task is done more efficiently and faster. Most importantly, when I commit to undivided attention to the present moment activity, I fully remember the details of the event. This one hour a day exercise is my antidote to improve my memory.

Multitasking is so widely accepted in our society that it is a habit hard to break. If you want to experiment with this exercise, it is best to start with a designated time. With this heightened concentration, you will have better recall. When you find your memory improving, you might want to make this exercise a way of life.

The other day, I happened to see my friend Deana who recently lost her mother. Deana and I started talking about the caregiving responsibility that daughters especially take on for their aging parents. We also discussed how our lives are interrupted when this occurs.

During this conversation, Deana made a comment that I found extremely thought-provoking.

She said, "In the big scheme of life, it really is only a short time that our parents are in need of our caregiving. Instead of feeling that this is an interruption in our lives, it should be a time of enjoying the final years we have together. We certainly miss them when they are gone."

This is so true.

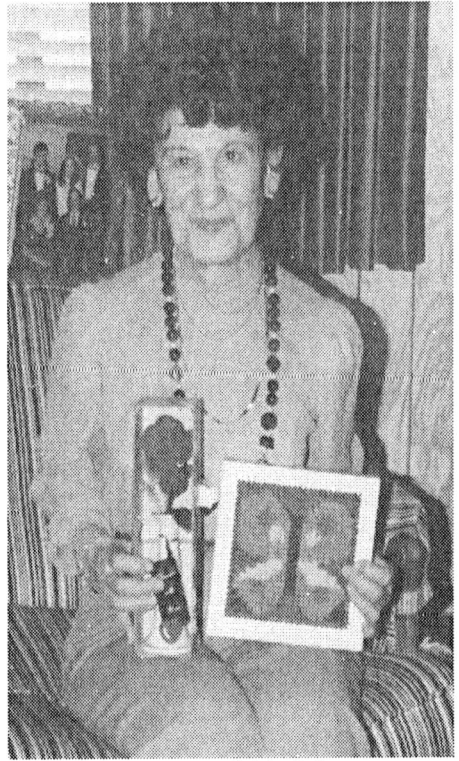

Mom at 75ᵗʰ birthday

Endnotes

[1] "Alzheimer's Disease Statistics, Alzheimer's disease in the United States," Alzheimer's Association (Fact sheet 2004) 1.

[2] Ibid.

[3] Ibid.

[4] "What Is PET," SNM, http://interactive.snm.org/index.cfm?PageID=972&RID=1307, accessed July 26, 2005.

[5] Non-invasive MRI Technique Distinguishes Between Alzheimer's And Frontotemporal Dementia,adapted from news release, University of California - San Francisco, http://www.sciencedaily.com/print.php?url=/releases/2005/06/050618160238.htm, accessed August 8, 2005.

[6] "New Test is First Step in Early Detection of Alzheimer's Disease," http.//www.alzheimersupport.com/library/showarticle.cfm/ID/2175/, accessed July 26,2005.

[7] Christine Kennard, Alzheimer Vaccine Follow-up Results Reported, Mild to Modrate Alzheimer's May Respond to Vaccine Therapy, http.//alzheimers.about.com/od/research/a/vaccine_follow.htm, accessed Aug. 23, 2005.

[8] Alzheimer Letter, Reagan, http://www.pbs.org/wgbh/amex/reagan/filmmore/reference/primary/alzheimers.html, accessed July 2005.

[9] "Alzheimer's Disease Statistics, Alzheimer's disease in the United States," Alzheimer's Association (fact sheet 2004)1.

[10] Ibid.

[11] M. Sano et al., "A Controlled Trial of Selegeline, Alpha-Tocopherol, or Both as Treatment for Alzheimer's Disease," *New England Journal of Medicine* 336 (1997): 1216-1222. http://content.nejm.org/cgi/content/full/336/17/1216, accessed July 18, 2005.

[12] High-ORAC Foods May Slow Aging, Recommendation For ORAC Consumption, http://www.discount-vitamins-herbs.net/ORAC.htm, accessed August 2, 2005.

[13] High-ORAC Foods May Slow Aging, *Agricultural Research Service, USDA* February 8, 1999.
http://www.aaccnet.org/FuncFood/content/releases/PR-High%20ORAC.htm, accessed August 3, 2005.

[14] R.I. Prior, "Antioxidant Capacity and Polyphenolic Components of Teas: Implications for Altering In Vivo Antioxidant Status," *Proceedings of the Society for Experimental Biology and Medicine* 220, no. 4 (1999): 255-261. Carper, *Your Miracle Brain:* 165.

[15] Anti Aging Library, Red Wine Molecule May Protect Brain from Alzheimer's, The World Health, http://www.worldhealth.net/p/230,4937.html, accessed August 26, 2005.

[16] Allison Stewart, "Chocolate Shown to Combat Aging," *Consumer Health Journal*, February 2004, http://www.consumerhealthjournal.com/articles/chocolate.htm, accessed August 6, 2005.

[17] S. Frautschy, The Curry Spice Curcumin Reduces Oxidative Damage and Amyloid Pathology in an Alzheimer Transgenic Mouse, *Journal of Neuroscience*, November 1, 2001, http://www.jneurosci.org/cgi/content/full/21/21/8370, accessed July 7, 2005.

[18] D. Snowdon, *Aging With Grace* (New York: Bantam, 2001): 173.

[19] Ibid, 179.

[20] Snowdon, Aging With Grace: 38.

[21] R.P. Friedland et al., "Patients with Alzheimer's disease have reduced activities in midlife compared with healthy control-group members," *Proceedings of National Academy of Sciences*, http://www.pnas.org/cgi/content/full/98/6/3440?maxtoshow=&HITS=10&hits=10&RESU.

[22] E.L. Helkala et al., "Midlife Vascular Risk Factors and Alzheimer's Disease in Later Life: Longitudinal Population-Based Study," *British Medical Journal* 322 (2001): 1447-1451.

[23] S. Seiner, "High Blood Pressure and High Cholesterol In Midlife May Increase Risks of Alzheimer's Disease," Vertitas

Medicine for Patients, Viewpoint on Alzheimer's Disease www.veritasmedicine.com/read_newsletter.cfm?vip=1-1-1&edition=125, accessed July 17, 2005.

[24] "Cholesterol: A Clue to Alzheimer's?" HealthAtoZ.com, http://www.healthatoz.com/atoz/Atoz/dc/caz/neur/alzh/alert11022000.jsp, accessed July 18, 2005.

[25] B. Wolozin et al., "Decreased Prevalence of Alzheimer's Disease Associated with 3-Hydroxy-3- methyglutaryl Coenzyme A Reductase Inhibitors," *Archives of Neurology* 57 (2000): 1439.

[26] Snowden, *Aging with Grace*: 95.

[27] Ibid., 193-194

[28] "Risk factors and prevention strategies," Health AtoZ, http://www.healthatoz.com/healthatoz/Atoz/dc/caz/neur/alzh/alert11022000.jsp, accessed July 18, 2005.

[29] D.H.Smith, "Long-Term Accumulation of Amyloid-B in Axons Following Brain Trauma Without Persistent Upregulation of Amyloid Precursor Protein Genes," *Journal of Neuropathology & Experimental Neurology* vol. 61, (No. 12): 1056-1068. http://neur.allenpress.com/neuronline/?request=get-document&issn=0022-3069&volume=, accessed July 18, 2005.

[30] "Education May Protect Against Alzheimer's Disease and Other Forms of Dementia," reporting on a study presented at the World Alzheimer's Disease Congress 2000 by Margaret Gatz, Ph.D., professor of psychology at the University of Southern California, Los Angeles, Alzheimer's Association. www.alz.org/Media/newsreleases/2000/07090Research.asp, accessed July 18, 2005.

[31] Friedland et al., *Proceedings of National Academy of Sciences.*

[32] Brett Foley, "Too much Television linked to dementia, *The Age* 3 July 2001 Section: News 3. http://newsstore.fairfax.com.au/apps/viewDocument.ac?multiview=true&sy=age&page=1, accessed July 7, 2005.

[33] "Alzheimer's Disease and Related Dementias in Pennsylvania: A Growing Crisis, A Model For Change," Alzheimer's Association Pennsylvania Public Policy Coalition. 4.

[34] Ibid.

[35] R.J. Hodes, V.Cahan, M. Pruzan, "The National Institute on Aging at the Twentieth Anniversary: Achievements and Promise of Research on Aging," *Journal of American Geriatrics Society* 44, no. 2 (1996): 204-6. http://www.ncbi.nlm.nih.gov, accessed July 29, 2005.

[36] "Impact on Society About Alzheimer's Disease, Alzheimer's Association (fact sheet 2004) 2.

[37] "Causes of Alzheimer's disease," About Alzheimer's disease, Alzheimer's Association (fact sheet 2004) 1.

[38] "Worldwide cost of Alzheimer's disease and dementia estimated at $156 billion," Alzheimer's Association International Conference on Prevention of Dementia, Alzheimer's Association, June 20, 2005 in Washington DC. http://www.alz.org/preventionconference/pc2005/062005costAd.asp, accessed July 18, 2005.

[39] Ibid.

Printed in the United States
47946LVS00003B/109-144